Challenging Behaviour

Third Edition

Challenging Behaviour

Third Edition

Eric Emerson

Professor of Disability and Health Research, Lancaster University, Lancaster, UK, and Visiting Professor, Australian Family and Disability Studies Research Collaboration, University of Sydney, Sydney, Australia.

Stewart L. Einfeld

Chair of Mental Health, Faculty of Health Sciences, and Senior Scientist, Brain and Mind Research Institute, University of Sydney, Sydney, Australia.

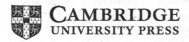

CAMBRIDGE
UNIVERSITY PRESS

University Printing House, Cambridge CB2 8BS, United Kingdom

Cambridge University Press is part of the University of Cambridge.

It furthers the University's mission by disseminating knowledge in the pursuit of education, learning and research at the highest international levels of excellence.

www.cambridge.org
Information on this title: www.cambridge.org/9780521728935

First edition published by Cambridge University Press 1995
Second edition published by Cambridge University Press 2001
Third edition published by Cambridge University Press 2011
3rd printing 2014

A catalogue record for this publication is available from the British Library

Library of Congress Cataloguing in Publication data
Emerson, Eric, 1953–
Challenging behaviour / Eric Emerson, Stewart L. Einfeld. – 3rd ed.
    p. cm.
Includes bibliographical references and index.
ISBN 978-0-521-72893-5 (pbk.)
1. People with mental disabilities – Mental health.   2. People with mental disabilities – behavior modification.   I. Einfeld, Stewart L.   II. Title.
RC451.4.M47E44   2011
362.196´89–dc22

                                                                      2010037292

ISBN 978-0-521-72893-5 Paperback

....

To the memory of Edward G (Ted) Carr (1947–2009),
an inspiring leader.

Contents

Chapter 12 authored by:
David Allen
Associate Clinical Director, Directorate of Learning Disability Services, ABMUHB and Professor of Clinical Psychology in Learning Disability, Cardiff University, Cardiff, Wales

Introduction

Around 0.1% of people have a severe intellectual disability and also engage in 'challenging' behaviours such as aggression, self-injury and destructiveness. This combination of severe intellectual and behavioural disabilities can significantly limit the life experiences of the person themselves and can place the health, safety and welfare of those who support them in jeopardy. They also represent a significant challenge to organizations involved in providing educational, health and welfare supports for people with intellectual disabilities.

Over the past four decades we have learned much about the nature of challenging behaviours and have developed approaches to support and intervention that have been shown to be effective, for some people, in bringing about rapid and socially significant reductions in challenging behaviour. The primary aim of this book is to provide a concise overview of this body of knowledge. This is not, however, a 'how-to-do-it' book. Instead, it will focus on describing developments in knowledge that have important implications for practice. A range of alternative texts are available for those seeking detailed instructions for carrying out intervention programmes (Ball *et al.*, 2004; Clements and Zarkowska, 2000; Luiselli, 2006; McLean and Grey, 2007; Sigafoos *et al.*, 2003; Thompson, 2008; Woodward *et al.*, 2007).

Virtually all of the studies mentioned in this book have been undertaken in one of the world's richer countries, and more often than not in one of the world's richer English-speaking countries. This bias reflects the existing pattern of inequalities in investment in health and social research related to people with intellectual disability (Emerson *et al.*, 2007a). However, we believe that many of the basic processes that underlie challenging behaviours are likely to be relatively universal and, as such, transcend cultural boundaries. What is culturally specific, however, is knowledge that relates to the organization and effectiveness of services designed to support people with intellectual disabilities and challenging behaviours. As such, the latter chapters of this book may be more relevant in some countries than others.

Terms and definitions

Intellectual disability

The terms used to refer to people with intellectual disabilities have undergone numerous changes over the last century. As terms used to describe socially devalued groups enter the common vocabulary, they quickly acquire disparaging connotations. Today's scientific terminology quickly becomes tomorrow's terms of abuse. 'Idiots', 'imbeciles', 'morons', 'subnormals' and 'retards' are nowadays nothing more than terms of denigration. In this chapter we use the term intellectual disability in preference to the synonymous terms 'mental retardation', still used in the main psychiatric classificatory systems and in many countries around the world (American Psychiatric Association, 2000; World Health Organization, 1992, 1996, 2007), and 'learning disability' (often used in health and social care systems in the UK).

This choice reflects the emergence of intellectual disability as the preferred terminology within the international scientific community (cf., the International Association for the Scientific Study of Intellectual Disability, the American Association on Intellectual and Developmental Disabilities) (Harris, 2005). It also avoids the confusion arising from terms which have very different meanings in different countries (e.g. 'learning disability' has very different meanings in the UK and USA) and avoids the use of terms which in many countries have acquired disparaging connotations (e.g. mental handicap, mental retardation).

The definition of intellectual disability involves two core components: a general deficit in cognitive functioning, which emerges during childhood (American Psychiatric Association, 2000; Harris, 2005; World Health Organization, 1992, 1996). A 'general deficit in cognitive functioning' is usually taken as a score of less than two standard deviations below the mean on a standardized IQ test. Given that most IQ tests are constructed to have a mean of 100 and a standard deviation of 15, this is ordinarily equivalent to a score below 70. This aspect of the definition is important in discriminating between people with significant deficits in multiple areas of cognitive functioning and people with very specific cognitive deficits (or specific learning difficulties such as dyslexia). The second component of the definition (emergence during childhood, typically before the age of 18) is important in distinguishing people with intellectual disability from people with cognitive deficits acquired in later life; in particular, deficits associated with dementias.

A third component, that the person also shows deficits in adaptive behaviours or social functioning, is sometimes added to the definition. However, classificatory systems differ in the extent to which such deficits are seen as an inherent characteristic of the deficit in cognitive functioning or as an independent characteristic whose presence needs to be determined for the classification to apply. For example, the World Health Organization's ICD-10 guidance suggests that 'adaptive behaviour is *always impaired*, but in protected social environments where support is available this impairment may not be at all obvious in subjects with mild mental retardation' (World Health Organization, 1996). In contrast, adaptive behaviour is considered as an independent criteria in the commonly used definition advocated by the American Association on Intellectual and Developmental Disabilities (AIDD, formerly the American Association on Mental Retardation; AAMR) (Luckasson et al., 2002; Schalock et al., 2007).

Unlike the measurement of cognitive functioning, there is at present no consensus on how 'impairments' or 'deficits' in adaptive behaviour should be operationalized. Indeed, there is a strong scientific case for considering social functioning and adaptive behaviour as a possible outcome of the interaction between impaired cognitive ability and prevailing social arrangements (rather than as a defining characteristic of intellectual disability). Such an approach is consistent with the World Health Organization's International Classification of Functioning, Disability and Health (ICF) (World Health Organization, 2001; World Health Organization, 2007a). While the ICF recognizes the important association between impairments in 'intellectual functions' and disability, it does not include prescriptive cut-offs for such impairments.

Intellectual disability is often considered to comprise two distinct groups (Einfeld and Emerson, 2008). The first represents the lower end of the normal distribution of intelligence in the population. This group predominantly comprises individuals with mild intellectual disability that is presumed to result from both genetic and environmental influences. The second group comprises people whose 'general deficit in cognitive functioning' is the result of identifiable or apparent disorders, of genetic or environmental origin. In this group, intellectual disability is typically more severe and people are also much more likely to have other neurological problems such as epilepsy, sensory or motor deficits. Among people with severe intellectual disability, language may be absent or limited to individual words or phrases, or a limited range of signs may be used in communication.

Our concern within this book is primarily with people with severe intellectual disability. However, we will, at times, also draw on evidence and knowledge derived from studies of people with a wide range of intellectual disabilities. We will also draw on evidence and knowledge derived from studies of people who do not have intellectual disability.

Challenging behaviour

Over the two decades, the term 'challenging behaviour', initially promoted in North America by The Association for People with Severe Handicaps, has come to replace a number of related terms including abnormal, aberrant, disordered, disturbed, dysfunctional, maladaptive and problem behaviours. These terms have previously been used to describe broad classes of behaviours shown by people with severe intellectual disabilities. They include aggression, destructiveness, self-injury, stereotyped mannerisms and a range of other behaviours, which may be either harmful to the individual (e.g. eating inedible objects), challenging for carers and care staff (e.g. non-compliance, persistent screaming, disturbed sleep patterns, overactivity) and/or objectionable to members of the public (e.g. regurgitation of food, the smearing of faeces over the body).

The term challenging behaviour has been defined as 'culturally abnormal behaviour(s) of such an intensity, frequency or duration that the physical safety of the person or others is likely to be placed in serious jeopardy, or behaviour which is likely to seriously limit use of, or result in the person being denied access to, ordinary community facilities' (Emerson, 1995, 2001a) or as 'behaviour ... of such an intensity, frequency or duration as to threaten the quality of life and/or the physical safety of the individual or others and is likely to lead to responses that are restrictive, aversive or result in exclusion' (Royal College of Psychiatrists et al., 2007). There is little meaningful difference between these two definitions.

The term challenging behaviour will be used throughout the remainder of the book for a number of reasons. First, it is free from implicit assumptions regarding the characteristics of the behaviour. A number of alternative terms have unhelpful connotations regarding either the organization of behaviour (e.g. disordered behaviour) or the nature of the relationship between the behaviour and ongoing events (e.g. dysfunctional or maladaptive behaviour). As we shall see, considerable evidence suggests that for some people in some contexts 'challenging' behaviours may be both orderly and adaptive. Indeed, many challenging behaviours can be construed as (at least in the short term) coherently organized adaptive responses to 'challenging' situations.

Second, the term is specific to a socially significant sub-class of abnormal, odd or unusual behaviours. Challenging behaviour only refers to behaviours which involve significant risks to people's physical well-being or act to markedly reduce access to community settings. This consequently excludes behaviours which may be either statistically or culturally infrequent but have a less pronounced physical or social impact.

Culturally abnormal behaviours shown by people with severe intellectual disabilities which are likely to place the physical safety of the person or others in serious jeopardy include serious physical aggression, destructiveness and self-injury as well as such health-threatening behaviours as the smearing of faeces over the body and the eating of inedible objects. Less serious forms of physical and verbal aggression and, perhaps, minor self-injury and stereotypy are included in this definition because they may limit or prevent them gaining access to ordinary community facilities. In the main, however, the focus throughout this book will be on more seriously challenging behaviours.

It should be noted that challenging behaviour, as defined above, is not synonymous with psychiatric disorder. Not all psychiatric disorders (e.g.

anxiety, mild depression) place the safety of the person or others in jeopardy, or lead to the person being denied access to community settings. Nevertheless, there does exist a significant overlap between challenging behaviours and some categories of psychiatric disorder (e.g. conduct disorders in children). We will return to these issues later in the book.

Finally, the use of the term 'challenge' may help to focus our attention on the process by which social problems are created and defined. That is, it may help to broaden the focus of enquiry by placing individual 'pathology' in the social and interpersonal context in which certain acts are deemed problematic. As was pointed out over 20 years ago, the term challenging behaviour 'emphasizes that such behaviours represent challenges to services rather than problems which individuals with intellectual disabilities in some way carry around with them' (Blunden and Allen, 1987). Indeed, when the term was introduced, it was intended to emphasise that problems were often caused as much by the way in which a person was supported as by their own characteristics (Department of Health, 2007). Since then, there has been a drift towards using the term simply as a diagnostic label for people. This is both inappropriate and unhelpful (Department of Health, 2007; Royal College of Psychiatrists *et al.*, 2007). We will use the term in its original meaning in this book.

To construe a situation as a challenge rather than as a problem may encourage more constructive responses. However, it would, of course, be mistaken to believe that minor changes in terminology are capable of bringing about major changes in practice.

An overview

Our book is split into two main sections. The first section focuses on what has been learned to date regarding our understanding of challenging behaviours. In Chapter 2, **The social context of challenging behaviour**, some of the social processes that are involved in defining behaviour as challenging will be highlighted and some of the personal and social consequences that arise from having a severe intellectual disability and challenging behaviour will be examined. Throughout these discussions it will be argued that challenging behaviour must be seen as a social construction. The implications of this perspective will then be explored in relation to approaches to assessing the impact of interventions and supports. In the following chapter, **Epidemiology**, we will look at the available evidence regarding the prevalence, incidence and natural history of challenging behaviours. This information will add to our understanding of the social significance of challenging behaviour. In addition, we will review the results of research that has attempted to identify factors which place people at risk of developing challenging behaviour. Such information may give some insight into the types of processes that may underlie challenging behaviours. It is also of potential value in targeting approaches to the prevention of challenging behaviour.

The following three chapters summarize the results of three quite distinct approaches to investigating the processes believed to possibly underlie challenging behaviours. In this series of chapters we will move from biological, through behavioural, to consideration of broader social processes. In Chapter 4, **Biological models and behavioural phenotypes**, we will review the burgeoning evidence relating to genetic and biological processes associated with challenging behaviours. In Chapter 5, **Behavioural models**, the models and concepts that underlie modern applied behavioural approaches to analysis and intervention will be discussed. In Chapter 6, **Social determinants**, we will turn to consider some of the wider social determinants of challenging behaviours. In the final chapter in this section, **An integrated approach**, we will explore possible linkages and associations between these very different approaches to understanding challenging behaviours.

The second section of the book focuses on the design and implementation of interventions and supports for people with severe intellectual disability and challenging behaviours. In Chapter 8, **The bases of intervention**, we will consider some of the broad perspectives and issues that should guide all approaches to intervention. In the following chapter, **Assessment and formulation**, we will review current knowledge and practice regarding the assessment of challenging behaviours from both biological and behavioural perspectives. The following two chapters will address current knowledge regarding the efficacy and effectiveness of **Psychopharmacological approaches** and **behavioural approaches** to intervention. Chapter 12, **The situational management of challenging behaviour** (written by David Allen), will address a related issue, approaches to the effective management, containment and diffusion of episodes of challenging behaviours.

The final chapter of the book turns to more general issues. In particular, we argue the case for taking a broader 'public health' approach to the issue of challenging behaviours, an approach that includes a significantly greater investment in preventative interventions.

2

The social context of challenging behaviour

We have defined challenging behaviour as *culturally abnormal behaviour* of such an intensity, frequency or duration that the physical safety of the person or others is likely to be placed in serious jeopardy, *or behaviour that is likely to seriously limit use of, or result in the person being denied access to, ordinary community facilities* (Emerson, 1995). This amendment to an earlier definition (Emerson *et al.*, 1988) made explicit the importance of social and cultural expectations and norms in defining behaviour as challenging.

Challenging behaviour is a social construction. Whether a behaviour is defined as challenging in a particular context will be dependent upon such factors as:

- social rules regarding what constitutes appropriate behaviour in that setting;
- the ability of the person to give a plausible account for their behaviour;
- the beliefs held by other participants in the setting about the nature of intellectual disabilities and the causes of the person's 'challenging' behaviour;
- capacity within the setting to manage any social disruption caused by the person's behaviour.

Behaviour in social settings is, at least in part, governed by implicit and explicit rules and expectations regarding what constitute appropriate conduct. The more formal the setting, the more explicit the rules. Indeed, context is essential in giving meaning to any behaviour. Behaviour can only be defined as challenging in particular contexts. For example, loud shouting and the use of 'offensive' language are likely to be tolerated (if not actually condoned) in restaurant kitchens and at football (soccer) matches. The same behaviour would certainly be considered 'challenging' during most religious services. Physical aggression is positively valued in the boxing ring. Severe self-directed aggression, is likely to be seen as challenging when shown by a person with intellectual disabilities, but may be viewed as a mark of religious piety when shown by a flagellant. At a more mundane level, stereotypic rocking is less likely to be tolerated in public places than in an institution for people with intellectual disabilities or in a nightclub.

Challenging Behaviour, 3rd edn, ed. Eric Emerson and Stewart L. Einfeld. Published by Cambridge University Press. © E. Emerson and S. L. Einfeld 2011.

Expectations concerning the appropriateness of particular behaviours are also determined by cultural beliefs and general role expectations. Supporting a young man to enjoy a beer in the local pub may be seen as a positive achievement by young white staff in a residential service for people with intellectual disabilities, as unremarkable by other customers in the local pub, and as highly problematic by the young man's devout Muslim family. Similarly, physical aggression may be seen as being more deviant (in terms of involving a greater discrepancy between performance and cultural expectations) when shown by a woman with intellectual disabilities than when shown by a man.

As well as transgressing social conventions, people with disabilities are also likely to be cast in deviant or abnormal social roles. These may serve to modify the operation of contextual rules which ascribe meaning to behaviour. Thus, for example, viewing people with intellectual disabilities as 'eternal children' (Wolfensberger, 1972, 1975) may help absolve the person of personal responsibility for being challenging. In a similar vein, if a person is labelled as having an intellectual disability, observers will tend to ascribe their success on a task to external factors (e.g. the simplicity of the task), while ascribing failure to internal factors such as the person's cognitive impairments (Severence and Gastrom, 1977).

These processes may have a number of consequences, including increased tolerance for odd or deviant behaviour as long as the person is clearly identified as belonging to a defined group for whom personal responsibility is reduced. Indeed, the expectations surrounding group membership may include a positive expectation that the person will behave in unusual or odd ways. So, for example, members of the public may show greater tolerance for stereotypic rocking when shown by a person whom they can clearly label as having an intellectual disability than they would of an 'ordinary' member of the public.

The capacity of a setting to cope with any disruption caused by a person's challenging behaviour is also likely to contribute to determining whether they will be excluded. So, for example, the increased pressure in the UK on mainstream schools to demonstrate academic achievement is likely to increase the pressure to exclude pupils with intellectual disabilities who show challenging behaviour (Mental Health Foundation, 1997). Fluctuations in the levels of experience, competence, stress, stability and fatigue among members of a staff team are likely to determine their capacity to cope with the disruption caused by someone who shows severe self-injury.

Of course, none of these factors is static. The social acceptability of particular behaviours changes over time within and across cultures (e.g. the reduced tolerance of smoking in public places in the UK and North America). Expectations and norms governing behaviour within settings vary over time and across locations. As has been discussed above, the capacity of settings to manage the social disruption caused by challenging behaviour is likely to be influenced by factors ranging from public policy to local fluctuations in staff sickness.

While contextual factors are crucial to defining behaviour as challenging, it would be surprising if there were no commonalities between people and settings in their tendency to perceive particular behaviours as more or less challenging. For example, Lowe and Felce summarized the results of two studies that suggested that the level of social disruption caused by a behaviour was integral to its definition as 'challenging' by carers and care staff (Lowe and Felce, 1995a; Lowe and Felce, 1995b). In the first study, analysis of carer and staff ratings collected over a 4-year period on 92 people with intellectual disabilities indicated that behaviours that caused the greatest social disruption (e.g. aggression) or had significant implications for the duty of care exercised by carers or care staff (e.g. running away) were rated as creating the most challenging. In the second study, they reported that the probability of referral to specialized challenging behaviour services was significantly increased if the person showed high levels of behaviours that were likely to be socially disruptive (e.g. aggression, non-compliance).

Similarly, Kiernan and Kiernan employed discriminant function analysis to identify factors which distinguished 'more difficult' from 'less difficult pupils' with severe intellectual disabilities in a survey of segregated special schools in England and Wales (Kiernan and Kiernan, 1994). The first ten factors, in order of significance for pupils without mobility limitations, were: physical aggression involving significant risk to others; persistent interruption of activities of other pupils; social disruption (e.g. screaming); violent temper tantrums occurring weekly; unpredictability of challenging behaviour; breakage of windows, fixtures and fittings; aggression toward other pupils; lack of understanding of emotions of others; non-compliance.

Consideration of the range of social issues involved in defining behaviour as challenging is important for a number of reasons. First, it highlights the importance of explicitly acknowledging the operation of such factors in the definition of challenging behaviour, including operational definitions of challenging behaviour employed in epidemiological research. Unless we acknowledge the importance of social and cultural factors in defining challenging behaviour, we may be tempted to search for ever more refined mechanical and physical definitions of an inherently social process. Such a course of action would, of course, be doomed to failure.

Second, viewing challenging behaviour as a social construction illustrates the complexity of the phenomenon and helps to begin to identify some possible approaches to intervention. Thus, for example, if a person's minor stereotypy has been defined as challenging primarily due to the avoidance behaviours it elicits in others, in some situations intervention may be most appropriately aimed at reducing such avoidance, rather than eliminating stereotypy.

Finally, conceptualizing challenging behaviour as a complex social phenomenon, rather than simply a problem of aberrant behaviour, has considerable implications for evaluating the social significance of the outcomes of intervention. Prior to discussing this point in more detail, it is useful to examine what is known about the social impact of challenging behaviours.

The impact of challenging behaviours

The social significance of challenging behaviours is determined by the interaction of two factors. First, as we shall see in the next chapter, a significant minority of people with intellectual disabilities show challenging behaviours. Second, such behaviours are often associated with a range of negative personal and social consequences.

By definition, seriously challenging behaviours may significantly impair the health and/or quality of life of the person themselves, those who care for them and those who live or work with them. Self-injurious behaviours can result in damage to the person's health through secondary infections, malformation of the sites of repeated injury through the development of calcified haematomas, loss of sight or hearing, additional neurological impairments and even death. Similarly, serious aggression may result in significant injury to others as well as to the person themselves as a result of the defensive or restraining action of others (Allen et al., 2006; Allen, 2008; Jones et al., 2007; Konarski et al., 1997).

However, the consequences of challenging behaviours go far beyond their immediate physical impact. Indeed, the combined responses of the public, carers, care staff and service agencies to people who show challenging behaviours may prove significantly more detrimental to their quality of life than the immediate physical consequences of the challenging behaviours themselves. These social responses may include abuse, inappropriate treatment, social exclusion, deprivation and systematic neglect.

Abuse

It is, perhaps, not surprising that the difficulties involved in caring for people with challenging behaviours and, in particular, the management of episodes of challenging behaviour, may, at times, lead to inappropriate reactions from carers and care staff. Some of these reactions include physical abuse. Thus, for example, challenging behaviour has been identified as a major predictor of documented instances of abuse in a North American institutional setting (Rusch et al., 1986). Remarkably, 1 in 40 ward staff in Montreal institutions for people with intellectual disabilities indicated that their typical response to an episode of self-injury was to hit the resident (Maurice and Trudel, 1982).

Inappropriate treatment

Challenging behaviours have often been 'managed' by methods of control, some of which can be considered detrimental to the well-being of the person themselves (Department of Health, 2007; Royal College of Psychiatrists *et al.*, 2007). Studies undertaken in North America and the UK suggest that, in many localities, approximately one in two people with severe intellectual disabilities who show challenging behaviours are prescribed anti-psychotic medication (Davidson *et al.*, 1994; Emerson *et al.*, 2000; Kiernan *et al.*, 1995; Robertson *et al.*, 2000; Robertson *et al.*, 2005).

Such a widespread use of anti-psychotic medication raises a number of concerns as: (1) there is little evidence that anti-psychotics have any specific effect in reducing challenging behaviours; (2) such medication has a number of well documented serious side effects; and (3) the use of anti-psychotics can be substantially reduced through peer review processes with no apparent negative effects for the majority of participants (Ahmed *et al.*, 2000; Davis *et al.*, 1998). As has been pointed out, while the results of drug reduction programmes 'are heartening, they suggest that much of the medication was unnecessary when either originally prescribed or by the time the reduction programme was instituted' (Singh and Repp, 1989) (see also Chapter 10).

Similarly, the use of mechanical restraints and protective devices to manage self-injury gives cause for serious concern. Such procedures can lead to muscular atrophy, demineralization of bones and shortening of tendons as well as resulting in other injuries during the process of the restraints being applied (Jones *et al.*, 2007; Luiselli, 1992). Finally, people with severe intellectual disabilities have historically been at significant risk of exposure to unnecessarily degrading or abusive psychological treatments (G. Allen Roeher Institute, 1988; Repp and Singh, 1990).

Social exclusion, deprivation and systematic neglect

Challenging behaviours are a major cause of stress experienced by parents (Hastings, 2002) and have been associated, among other factors, with families' decisions to seek an out-of-home residential placement for their son or daughter (Llewellyn *et al.*, 2005; Tausig, 1985). Children and adults with challenging behaviours are significantly more likely to be excluded from community-based services and to be admitted, re-admitted to or retained in more remote and more institutional settings (Department of Health, 2007; Emerson and Robertson, 2008; Perry *et al.*, 2007; Royal College of Psychiatrists *et al.*, 2007). Once admitted to institutional care they commonly spend much of their time in materially deprived surroundings, disengaged from their world and avoided by staff (Mansell, 1995). Within community-based settings, challenging behaviours may serve to limit the development of social relationships, reduce opportunities to participate in community-based activities and employment, and prevent access to health and social services (Anderson *et al.*, 1992; Beadle-Brown *et al.*, 2005; Hill and Bruininks, 1984; Jacobsen *et al.*, 1984; Martorell *et al.*, 2008; Robertson *et al.*, 2001a).

Finally, people who show challenging behaviours are unlikely to receive effective support for their challenging behaviours (Emerson *et al.*, 2000; Emerson, 2001b). Thus, for example, an investigation of treatment and management practices among 265 people with challenging behaviours receiving some form of residential support reported that only 15% of participants had a written behaviourally orientated treatment programme (Emerson *et al.*, 2000). Given the evidence that now exists in support of the use of such treatment approaches (see Chapter 11), these data highlight a glaring failure in the extent to which services for people with severe intellectual disability embody the principle of 'evidence-based practice'.

Summary

The above sections illustrate some of the negative ways in which challenging behaviours may shape the lives of people with severe intellectual disability and those who support them. It is important to keep in mind, however, that these are not inevitable consequences that are inherent to the phenomena of challenging behaviour. Rather, they are associations which have arisen in particular service systems located in particular cultures at particular points in time. While, as mentioned in the previous chapter, it would be surprising if there were no commonalities between social responses to challenging behaviour in high income English-speaking countries, it is important that we keep in mind that these consequences result from the ways in which service systems support (or fail) people with challenging behaviour. For example, we undertook a series of multivariate analyses to identify personal and environmental characteristics associated with variation in the quality of life among people receiving community-based residential supports from agencies nominated as proving examples of better practice. This analyses failed to identify any significant relationship between the severity of challenging behaviour shown by participants and their quality of life in such areas as self-determination, contact with members of their family, social inclusion, employment, physical activity, risk and community participation (Emerson *et al.*, 1999c; Robertson *et al.*, 2001a; Robertson *et al.*, 2001b).

Intervention outcomes

Over the past three decades people have paid increasing attention to the importance of measuring and monitoring the outcomes of interventions, services and supports. But what outcomes should be measured? Traditionally, the success of interventions or services for people with challenging behaviour has been rather mechanistically judged against their effectiveness in reducing the frequency, duration or severity of challenging behaviour. These are, of course, relevant outcomes. But are they sufficient?

The notion of 'social validity' was introduced into behavioural practice in the late 1970s. An intervention can be considered to be socially valid if it addresses a socially significant problem (such as challenging behaviour), but in a manner which is acceptable to the main stakeholders involved (and therefore avoids the use of abusive or degrading procedures) and results in *outcomes that are important to the main stakeholders involved* (Kazdin and Matson, 1981; Wolf, 1978). At the same time, Evans and Meyer (1985) have argued the case for expanding current practice to include the assessment of the 'meaningful outcomes' of intervention (Evans and Meyer, 1985; Meyer and Janney, 1989; Meyer and Evans, 1993) such as:

- the targeted challenging behaviour and other challenging behaviours shown by the person;
- replacement skills and behaviours, including, for example, the development of self-control strategies to support behaviour change and the development of alternative communicative responses;
- procedures for managing the person's challenging behaviour including use of medication, restraint and crisis management techniques;
- health-related consequences of the person's challenging behaviour such as trauma, skin irritations;
- the restrictiveness of the person's residential and vocational placement;
- broader aspects of the person's quality of life including physical and social integration, personal life satisfaction, affect and the range of choices available to the individual;
- the perceived significance of the person's challenging behaviour by others (e.g. family, staff, public).

Building on these developments, Fox and Emerson attempted to identify the outcomes of intervention which were considered particularly salient by a number of stakeholder groups (including people with intellectual disability, parents of people with intellectual disability, professionals, managers and direct support workers) and then develop a simple tool to help people identify and measure relevant outcomes (Fox and Emerson, 2001, 2002, in press). The results of this project indicated that reduction in the severity of challenging behaviour was considered the most important outcome of intervention by approximately half of the stakeholder groups. Other outcomes considered to be the most important by stakeholder groups included increased friendships and relationships, changes in the perceptions of individuals by others, the person learning alternative ways of getting their needs met, increased control and empowerment. While there were high levels of agreement on the relative importance of outcomes between stakeholder groups who did not have an intellectual disability, levels of agreement between people with intellectual disability and all other stakeholder groups were poor.

This suggests that any attempt to evaluate the successes and failures of behavioural, or any other, approaches to intervention will need to take into account the range of outcomes which are of significance to the major stakeholders in the intervention process. The importance of such a multi-faceted approach to evaluating the impact of intervention is, in many ways, self-evident once the significance of social processes in the definition and response to challenging behaviour has been recognized. For example, can an intervention be considered successful if it reduces the rate of a person's self-injury by 75%, but still leaves them at high risk of losing their sight, being mechanically and psychopharmacologically restrained and subject to extensive social exclusion? We will return to these issues in Chapters 9 and 11.

3

The epidemiology of challenging behaviour

In this chapter we will address a number of issues that relate to the epidemiology of challenging behaviour. These include:

- the percentage and number of people with intellectual disabilities who show challenging behaviour;
- the prevalence of particular forms of challenging behaviour;
- the co-occurrence of different forms of challenging behaviour;
- personal and environmental risk factors associated with showing challenging behaviour;
- the emergence and persistence of challenging behaviour.

Epidemiological studies of challenging behaviours have focused, almost exclusively, on attempting to identify the *prevalence* of particular behaviours and investigate the relationship between prevalence and personal or environmental risk factors. That is, they have attempted to identify the number of individuals in the population under study (e.g. the total population of Lancaster) who, at a given point in time, show challenging behaviour and, through the use of correlational methods, to identify those personal and environmental characteristics associated with people being at increased risk of exhibiting these behaviours.

Prevalence rates vary as a function of the incidence and duration (or persistence) of a particular characteristic. *Incidence* is a measure of the number of new 'cases' appearing within a given population within a specified period of time (e.g. number of live births per year of children with Down syndrome in Lancaster, number of people *developing* self-injurious behaviour per year in Cardiff). *Persistence* (or duration) is a measure of the length of time a particular condition is present (e.g. the average number of days flu lasts, the average number of years a person will show self-injurious behaviour).

The prevalence of challenging behaviours

In the preceding chapter we stressed the importance of social processes and conditions in leading to particular behaviours being seen as challenging. One

Challenging Behaviour, 3rd edn, ed. Eric Emerson and Stewart L. Einfeld. Published by Cambridge University Press. © E. Emerson and S. L. Einfeld 2011.

implication of this approach is that attempts to measure the prevalence of challenging behaviour are themselves bound by the constraints and expectations of particular contexts and cultures. Estimates of the prevalence of challenging behaviour will also, of course, be influenced by such methodological factors as the selection of operational definitions, methods of case identification (e.g. review of case notes vs. interview with care staff) and the overall sampling strategy adopted within the study (e.g. total administratively defined population of people with intellectual disabilities, children with intellectual disabilities at school).

Relatively few studies have attempted to identify the prevalence of multiple forms of challenging behaviour among all people with intellectual disabilities in the total population living in a defined geographical area. More commonly, studies have focused on determining the prevalence of specific forms of challenging behaviour (e.g self-injurious behaviour) or have restricted sampling to specific sub-populations of people with intellectual disabilities (e.g. those living in institutional settings, community settings or children attending schools).

Total population studies

Total population studies attempt to measure the prevalence of challenging behaviour among *all* people with intellectual disabilities living in a particular community. This is a particularly difficult undertaking as administrative records of people with intellectual disabilities (e.g. local or national registers, lists of people who make use of services for people with intellectual disabilities) typically miss the majority of young children and adults with mild or moderate intellectual disabilities. We are not aware of any studies that have specifically addressed the prevalence of *challenging behaviour* in total population samples. There are, however, a small number of studies that have attempted to ascertain the prevalence of *behavioural difficulties or conduct disorders* among children with (and without) intellectual disabilities in representative national total population samples. The results of these studies have been very consistent in showing significantly increased rates of behavioural difficulties or conduct disorders among children with intellectual disabilities when compared with their peers. For example:

- Among 5–16-year-old British children, rates of formally diagnosable conduct disorders were 21% among children with intellectual disabilities, compared to 4% among children without intellectual disabilities (Emerson and Hatton, 2007d);
- Among 6–7-year-old Australian children, 24% of children with intellectual disabilities showed high levels of behavioural difficulties, compared to 8% of children without intellectual disabilities (Emerson *et al.*, 2010);

- Among 3-year-old British children, 30% of children with early cognitive delay showed high levels of behavioural difficulties, compared to 10% of children without early cognitive delay (Emerson and Einfeld, 2010)

Administrative population studies

More commonly, epidemiological studies have attempted to measure the prevalence of challenging behaviour in administratively defined populations of people with intellectual disabilities (e.g. children attending special schools, adult users of intellectual disabilities services) (Borthwick Duffy, 1994; Cooper et al., 2009a; Cooper et al., 2009b; Emerson et al., 2001a; Kiernan and Kiernan, 1994; Lowe et al., 2007). In one of the largest studies, Qureshi, Kiernan and colleagues conducted a survey in seven administrative areas in the North West of England with a total (general) population of 1.54 million (Kiernan and Qureshi, 1993; Qureshi and Alborz, 1992). They screened approximately 4200 people with intellectual disability, and identified people as showing serious challenging behaviours if they had:

- at some time caused more than minor injury to themselves or others, or destroyed their immediate living or working environment; or
- showed behaviours at least once a week that required the intervention of more than one member of staff to control, or placed them in danger, or caused damage which could not be rectified by care staff, or caused more than 1 hour's disruption;
- showed behaviours at least daily that caused more than a few minutes' disruption.

Using this definition, 1.91 people per 10 000 of the general population (range 1.41 to 2.55 per 10 000 across the seven areas) were identified as having an intellectual disability and serious challenging behaviour. This translates to an estimated prevalence rate of 6% of all people within these areas who had been administratively defined as having an intellectual disability. Since then other studies using identical or very similar methods have reported administrative prevalence rates of 3.33 and 3.62 per 10 000 of the general population (8% of the people with intellectual disabilities screened) in other areas in North West England (Emerson and Bromley, 1995; Emerson et al., 2001a).

Re-analysis of these data using a definition of 'more demanding' challenging behaviour gave rates of 4.6 (range 3.5–6.6) per 10 000, equivalent to approximately 10%–15% of people who had been administratively defined as having an intellectual disability (Emerson and Bromley, 1995; Emerson et al., 2001a; Kiernan et al., 1997). A more recent study undertaken across seven localities in Wales (total population 1.2 million) reported very similar prevalence rates of 4.5 (range 2.5–7.5) per 10 000 (Lowe et al., 2007).

However, markedly lower rates of 'more demanding' challenging behaviour (4% of people screened) have been reported in Norway (Holden and Gitlesen, 2006).

Types of challenging behaviours

Prevalence rates (in terms of the percentage of people administratively defined as having an intellectual disability) from the above studies for broad categories of challenging behaviour were: 2.1% physical aggression, 1.3% self-injury, 1.3% property destruction and 3.4% other forms of challenging behaviour. The use of other criteria can, of course, result in significantly greater prevalence rates. For example, use of the *Diagnostic Criteria for Psychiatric Disorders for Use with Adults with Learning Disabilities/Mental Retardation (DC-LD)* has been reported to give point prevalence rates of 9.8% for aggression and 4.9% for self-injury (Cooper *et al.*, 2009a; Cooper *et al.*, 2009b). Questionnaire-based studies can result in markedly higher rates (Crocker *et al.*, 2006; Tyrer *et al.*, 2006).

Of course, each of these broad groups of challenging behaviours is likely to contain a range of specific forms of, for example, self-injury. Studies which have focused on the prevalence of particular forms of challenging behaviour provide a more detailed breakdown of the specific behaviours contained in these general classes of challenging behaviours. For example, the most prevalent forms of aggression shown in the past month by 168 people with intellectual disabilities identified in one administratively defined area were: punching, slapping, pushing or pulling (51% of people showing aggression); kicking (24%); pinching (21%); scratching (20%); pulling hair (13%); biting (13%); head-butting (7%); using weapons (7%); choking, throttling (4%) (Harris, 1993). In a similar study, the most prevalent behaviours shown by 153 people with intellectual disabilities who showed aggression were: hitting others with their hands (75% of people showing aggression); verbal aggression (60%); hitting others with objects (41%); meanness or cruelty (34%); scratching (27%); pulling hair (23%); pinching (20%) and biting (16%) (Emerson *et al.*, 2001a).

The most common topographies of self-injurious behaviour shown by 596 people with intellectual disabilities identified through a survey carried out in south east England were: skin picking (39%); self-biting (38%); head punching/ slapping (36%); head to object banging (28%); body to object banging (10%); other (10%); hair removal (8%); body punching or slapping (7%); eye poking (6%); skin pinching (4%); cutting with tools (2%); anal poking (2%); other poking (2%); banging with tools (2%); lip chewing (1%); nail removal (1%); teeth banging (1%) (Oliver *et al.*, 1987). It should be noted that, in such studies, the totals usually add up to more than 100% due to the co-occurrence of different forms of challenging behaviour in the same individual, an issue which will be discussed in more detail below.

The co-occurrence of challenging behaviours

As has been indicated, people may show more than one form of challenging behaviour. Thus, in the Kiernan, Qureshi, Alborz, Emerson and Bromley series of studies, between one-half and two-thirds of people identified as showing challenging behaviour did so in two or more of the four possible areas (aggression, self-injury, property destruction and 'other' behaviour).

In addition to the co-occurrence of challenging behaviour across broadly defined categories, people are also likely to show multiple forms of challenging behaviour within categories. Thus, for example, in Oliver's study reported above 54% of the people identified as showing self-injurious behaviour engaged in more than one form of self-injury (Oliver *et al.*, 1987). Indeed, 3% (20 of the 596) engaged in five or more different forms of self-injury. This rose to 7% for people whose self-injury was managed by the use of protective devices (Murphy *et al.*, 1993).

Personal and environmental risk factors

One of the potentially significant contributions of epidemiological research is to identify those personal and environmental factors which are associated with variation in the prevalence of a particular disorder. The identification of such 'risk factors' may be useful in two ways. First, they may indicate the importance of possible causal mechanisms. Sir Richard Doll's identification of the association between smoking and lung cancer came from epidemiological study of risk factors for lung cancer. Second, if the associations between risk factors and a particular outcome are strong enough, they may allow the specific targeting of preventative interventions. Provided below, is a very brief summary of the evidence regarding some of the better established correlates of challenging behaviour among people with intellectual disabilities.

Gender

There is some evidence to suggest that boys and men are more likely to be identified as showing challenging behaviour than girls and women (Di Terlizzi *et al.*, 1999; Eyman and Call, 1977). This relationship may be more pronounced:
- for aggression and property destruction than for self-injury (Borthwick Duffy, 1994; Rojahn and Esbensen, 2002);

- in institutional settings (Qureshi, 1994);
- for more severe challenging behaviour (Kiernan and Kiernan, 1994).

It is important to note, however, that other studies have reported either little differences in rates by gender (Crocker *et al.*, 2006; Harris, 1993; Holden and Gitlesen, 2006; Lowe *et al.*, 2007) or higher rates of aggression among women with intellectual disabilities (Cooper *et al.*, 2009b).

Age

The prevalence of challenging behaviours appears to increase with age during childhood, reach a peak during the age range 15–34 and then decline (Borthwick Duffy, 1994; Holden and Gitlesen, 2006; Kiernan and Kiernan, 1994; Oliver *et al.*, 1987; Rojahn, 1994). When comparisons are made with the age structure of the total population of people with intellectual disabilities, it is apparent that challenging behaviours appear to be particularly over-represented in the 15–24 age group (Kiernan and Qureshi, 1993). However, when comparisons are made with the predicted age structure of the population of people with *severe* intellectual disabilities it appears that age-specific prevalence rates may not decline until late middle age (Emerson *et al.*, 2001a). These patterns are more complicated, however, when the prevalence of particular forms of challenging behaviour are examined. Oliver and colleagues, for example, report that, while multiple topographies, head to object banging, head punching and finger chewing are significantly more prevalent in younger people with self-injurious behaviour, skin picking and cutting with tools are more prevalent among older people (Oliver *et al.*, 1987).

Specific syndromes and disorders

An increase in the prevalence of some particular forms of challenging behaviour has been reported to occur in association with specific syndromes associated with intellectual disabilities (Dykens *et al.*, 2000; Harris, 2005). While these associations are discussed at greater length in Chapter 4, they include:

- self-injurious behaviour, specifically hand and lip biting, among *all* people who have Lesch–Nyhan syndrome;
- high prevalence of self-injurious hand-wringing in Rett syndrome;
- greater than expected prevalence of various forms of self-injurious behaviour in the Cornelia de Lange, Riley–Day and Fragile-X syndromes;
- greater than expected prevalence of hyperkinesis, attention deficits and stereotypy in Fragile-X syndrome;
- greater than expected prevalence of self-injury among people with autism spectrum disorders;
- high prevalence of challenging behaviours in Prader–Willi syndrome
- increased prevalence of challenging behaviour associated with epilepsy.

Level of intellectual impairment

In general, the prevalence of aggression, property destruction, self-injurious behaviour and other forms of challenging behaviours are positively correlated with degree of intellectual impairment (Borthwick Duffy, 1994; Cooper *et al.*, 2009a; Cooper *et al.*, 2009b; Holden and Gitlesen, 2006; Kiernan and Qureshi, 1993; Kiernan and Kiernan, 1994; Oliver *et al.*, 1987; Qureshi and Alborz, 1992; Qureshi, 1994; Rojahn and Esbensen, 2002). Thus, for example, in a Californian survey, 7% of people with mild intellectual disabilities, 14% of people with moderate intellectual disabilities, 22% of people with severe intellectual disabilities and 33% of people with profound intellectual disabilities showed one or more form of challenging behaviour (Borthwick Duffy, 1994). People with more severe intellectual impairment are also likely to show multiple forms of challenging behaviour (Borthwick Duffy, 1994; Oliver *et al.*, 1987).

Additional impairments

In addition to the overriding effects of level of intellectual impairment, challenging behaviours are more likely to be seen in people who:
● have additional impairments of vision or hearing (Cooper *et al.*, 2009a; Kiernan and Kiernan, 1994);
● are non-verbal or who have particular difficulty with receptive or expressive communication (Emerson *et al.*, 2001a; Holden and Gitlesen, 2006; Kiernan and Kiernan, 1994; Sigafoos, 2000);
● have poorer social skills (Duncan *et al.*, 1999);
● are reported to have periods of disturbed sleep (Kiernan and Kiernan, 1994);
● have mental health problems (Borthwick Duffy, 1994; Hemmings, 2007; Moss *et al.*, 2000).
Self-injury, in particular, is markedly more prevalent among people with severe intellectual disabilities who have significant impairments of mobility (Kiernan and Qureshi, 1993; Kiernan and Kiernan, 1994).

Setting

The prevalence of challenging behaviour is also positively related to living with paid carers and the level of restrictiveness in residential settings (Borthwick Duffy, 1994; Cooper *et al.*, 2009a; Cooper *et al.*, 2009b; Rojahn and Esbensen, 2002). For example, data from the Californian survey indicate that 3% of people living independently, 8% of people living with their families, 9% of people living in smaller (1–6 place) community facilities, 24% of people living in larger community-based facilities and 49% of people living in institutions were identified as showing one or more forms of challenging behaviour (Borthwick Duffy, 1994).

The interpretation of the relationship between setting and challenging behaviour is problematic as both severity of intellectual disability and severity of challenging behaviour are associated at increased risk of admission and re-admission to more restrictive settings. Indeed, since studies of the effects of deinstitutionalization have failed to identify any consistent effects of deinstitutionalization on challenging behaviour (Kozma *et al.*, 2009; Walsh *et al.*, 2008), it would appear that such behaviours lead to institutionalization, rather than institutional environments leading to challenging behaviour.

Summary

A number of interlinked personal and environmental characteristics have been associated with variations in the prevalence of challenging behaviour. Unfortunately, due to methodological limitations and the use of relatively simplistic approaches to analysis, it is rarely possible to identify the unique contribution made by individual factors. Hopefully, future research will help untangle this and other issues. Nevertheless, the existing data do provide a basis for beginning to identify populations most at risk and are suggestive of some possible underlying mechanisms, an issue to which we shall turn in the following chapters.

The natural history of challenging behaviours

As noted above, little is known about the natural history of challenging behaviours. The information which is available, however, suggests that seriously challenging behaviours are likely to have their onset in childhood and may be highly persistent over time.

Onset

A number of retrospective studies have reported that seriously challenging behaviours are likely to have their onset in childhood. Murphy and colleagues reported that the mean age of onset for people whose severe self-injurious behaviour was managed by protective devices was 7 years of age (Murphy *et al.*, 1993). Similarly, we have reported that, of the 29 individuals (mean age 28 years) identified by service agencies as being the 'most challenging', 27 had entered some form of institutional care (with an average age on admission of just 9.6 years); admissions often being for the same challenging behaviours they were displaying nearly two decades later (Emerson *et al.*, 1988).

More recently, Murphy and colleagues *et al.* (1999) followed up for 18 months a cohort of 17 young children (mean age at recruitment to the study, 5 years 7 months) who had been identified by teachers as *beginning* to show self-injury *in the previous three months* (Murphy *et al.*, 1999a). While as a group participants showed evidence of increased duration of self-injury over the study period, considerable variation was shown by individual participants. The only factor identified as being associated with the trajectory of the children's self-injury over time was the level of concern expressed by teachers at the onset of the study.

Persistence

Few studies have examined the course of challenging behaviour over time (Totsika and Hastings, 2009). Chris Kiernan and colleagues reported that 63% of 179 people identified as showing 'more demanding' challenging behaviour in a total population survey undertaken in 1987 were still showing 'more demanding' challenging behaviour when followed up 7 years later (Kiernan *et al.*, 1997). Persistence rates of approximately 80% over a 10-year period have also been reported by other investigators (Totsika *et al.*, 2008; Turner and Sloper, 1996). High rates of persistence of challenging behaviour have also been reported in pre-school children with developmental disabilities (Green *et al.*, 2005) and through childhood into adolescence (Chadwick *et al.*, 2005; Einfeld *et al.*, 2006).

A number of studies have examined the persistence of specific forms of challenging behaviour. Reported persistence rates for self-injury (in non-institutional settings) have included:

- 97% persistence over a 10-year period for people relocated from institutional to community settings (Windahl, 1988);
- 96% over a 2-year period (Murphy *et al.*, 1993);
- 84% over a 20-year period (Taylor *et al.*, under review)
- 75% over a 5-year period for young adults living with their families (Kiernan and Alborz, 1996);
- 71% over a 7 year follow-up period (Emerson *et al.*, 2001b)
- 62% over a 2-year period (Cooper *et al.*, 2009a).

Aggression and disruptive behaviours have also been reported to be highly persistent over time (Einfeld *et al.*, 2006; Eyman *et al.*, 1981; Leudar *et al.*, 1984; Reid and Ballinger, 1995), with reported persistence rates of 83% for aggression and 70% for destructive behaviour over a five year period for young adults living with their families (Kiernan and Alborz, 1996) and 72% among adults in community settings over a two year period (Cooper *et al.*, 2009b).

Very few studies have attempted to identify personal or environmental characteristics associated with variations in the persistence of challenging behaviours. Kiernan and colleagues reported that persistence of 'more demanding' challenging behaviour was associated with participants in 1988 showing: more severe challenging behaviour; more severe self-injurious behaviour (and specific topographies of self-injury); more frequent stereotypy; more severe intellectual disability; poorer communication skills, self-care skills and less ability to use money; lower ability to occupy themselves constructively or to behave appropriately in social situations (Kiernan *et al.*, 1997). The persistence of self-injurious behaviour in a sub-sample of this study was predicted by: site of injury (higher persistence being shown by people exhibiting head directed self-injury); reported (greater) stability of self-injury when first identified; and (younger) age (Emerson *et al.*, 2001b).

While there is evidence that interventions may bring about significant reductions in challenging behaviour over the short to medium term (see later chapters), evidence from long-term follow up studies indicates that such gains rarely involve the complete elimination of challenging behaviour and may require significant ongoing investment to sustain gains (Foxx, 1990; Jensen and Heidorn, 1993; Schroeder and MacLean, 1987).

While caution must be taken in extrapolating from such a restricted data base, the available evidence does suggest that severe challenging behaviours may be highly persistent *despite* relocation from specialized congregate care settings or significant changes in staffing resources and the quality of the physical environment (Kozma *et al.*, 2009; Walsh *et al.*, 2008). The possible persistence of challenging behaviours points to the need for services to develop the capacity to effectively manage the physical, personal and social consequences of severe self-injurious behaviours over considerable periods of time.

4

Biological influences

The previous chapters have concentrated on defining the social significance of challenging behaviour on the basis of its prevalence, persistence and the impact such behaviours may have on the person themselves and those who support them. Attention was also drawn to some of the personal and environmental risk factors that are associated with variation in the prevalence and, to a lesser extent, persistence of challenging behaviour. In the next four chapters we will turn our attention to trying to understand *why* a substantial minority of people with severe intellectual disability show challenging behaviour.

Behavioural and neurobiological/psychiatric traditions have dominated applied research within the field of intellectual disabilities. These approaches have generated voluminous amounts of basic and applied research, which have made significant contributions to our understanding of some of the mechanisms and processes that may underlie challenging behaviour. The more we understand about these processes, the greater our chances of developing effective ways of helping people overcome challenging behaviour. In this chapter we will summarize what is known about biological influences on challenging behaviour. In the following chapters we will summarize what is known about behavioural processes that may underlie challenging behaviour and the role of broader social influences on challenging behaviour. In Chapter 7 we will attempt to draw these disparate stands of knowledge together.

In order to develop effective behaviour management strategies for people with challenging behaviours, a broad-ranging assessment of factors contributing to the behaviour is needed. Such an assessment needs to consider potential factors within the individual and in their environment. Factors within the individual may be considered as products of their genetic and other physical health make-up, combined with the influence of their life experience.

This chapter describes some of the important aspects of health that may impact on behaviour. First, we describe some of the more common specific

Challenging Behaviour, 3rd edn, ed. Eric Emerson and Stewart L. Einfeld. Published by Cambridge University Press. © E. Emerson and S. L. Einfeld 2011.

genetic causes of intellectual disability that increase vulnerability to specific patterns of behaviour. This vulnerability is known as the behaviour phenotype of the disorder, a term analogous to the generally previous description of the physical phenotype. Then, we describe some of the psychiatric disorders of significant biological origin that may manifest in, or be associated with, challenging behaviours, followed by consideration of pain, epilepsy, side effects of psychotropic medications and temperament.

Behaviour phenotypes of genetic disorders

Fragile X syndrome

Fragile X syndrome is caused by an expansion of a trinucleotide sequence in the DNA in part of the X chromosome. This sequence is repeated about 30 times in normal individuals. In affected persons, the sequence is repeated 200–600 times. In carrier females, the sequence occurs 50–200 times (Hagerman and Hagerman, 2002). This disrupts the production of a protein called FMRP, which in turn results in the observed phenotype. Fragile X syndrome is the most common inherited cause of intellectual disability. The physical phenotype in Fragile X syndrome is characterized by a particular facial appearance, more obvious in affected adults. The face has a long shape with prominent ears. There are joint abnormalities with hyperextensibility common. In post-pubertal boys, the testes are enlarged. Epileptic seizures occur in some children, mainly resolving in adolescence. In males, around 50% have intellectual disability in the moderate or severe range, and about 30% are in the mild intellectual disability range. In females, 75% have normal IQ and 25% have mild intellectual disability. The degree correlates inversely to the level of FMRP (Loesch et al., 2004). However, children with Fragile X syndrome tend to decline in IQ score over time, but stabilize in adolescence (Fisch et al., 2002).

Fragile X boys have difficulty, compared with children with Down syndrome, in inhibiting repetition and in switching attention from one type of target to another (Wilding et al., 2002). Carrier females may show milder forms of this difficulty (Steyaert et al., 2003). Fragile X individuals have a number of characteristic behavioural and emotional disturbances. Self-injurious behaviour is common, noted in 58% of affected boys (Symons et al., 2003). Biting the back of the hand or fingers is the most commonly reported form of self-injury. Self-injurious behaviour is most likely to occur following the presentation of difficult task demands or changes in routine. Shyness and gaze avoidance are also behavioural features of Fragile X syndrome, occurring more frequently than in children with other causes of intellectual disability (Einfeld et al., 1999a). This observation led to the perception that Fragile X syndrome was a prominent cause of autism. However, further study showed that these behaviours are different from autism. The shyness and the gaze avoidance disappear with familiarity.

Intellectual disability is usually mild to moderate, and verbal intelligence often exceeds performance abilities in both affected males and non-learning disabled female carriers. The IQ may decline in childhood and adolescence with an average adult IQ in males in the low moderate range. Approximately 70% of females with the full mutation have an IQ less than 85. Verbal dyspraxia is common (Spinelli *et al.*, 1995).

Prader–Willi syndrome

Prader-Willi syndrome (PWS) is caused in over 50% of cases by a deletion of part of the long arm of chromosome 15 of paternal origin (Holland *et al.*, 2003). In other cases PWS is caused by uniparental maternal disomy, unbalanced translocations, or mutations of the imprinting centre of the same region of chromosome 15. PWS occurs in about one in 20 000 live births. The physical phenotype of PWS is characterized by hypotonia and feeding difficulties in infancy, then excessive appetite and obesity, sometimes extreme, hypogonadism, short stature, and small hands and feet in childhood. Individuals with PWS have abnormalities in hypothalamic function governing growth, appetite, temperature control, and sleep. Most individuals with PWS function in the mild intellectual disability range, but a few individuals have normal intelligence. Einfeld, *et al.* (1999b) compared a cohort of individuals with PWS with controls matched for age, gender and IQ on the Developmental Behavior Checklist DBC (Einfeld and Tonge, 1995). The behaviours significantly associated with PWS were: 'severe temper tantrums, e.g. stamps feet, slams doors'; 'gets obsessed with an idea or activity'; 'scratches or picks his/her skin'; 'eats non-food items, e.g. dirt, grass, soap'; 'gorges food. Will do anything to get food; e.g. takes food out of garbage bins or steals food'; and 'mood changes rapidly for no apparent reason'. The temper tantrums in PWS often have a rage-like quality. They are frequently, though not always, associated with food-seeking. Sometimes the rage attack may be indirectly associated with food. For example, a PWS child may be provoked to rage by perceiving that another child has been permitted easier access to food. There is evidence of hypothalamic disturbance from both postmortem and fMRI studies (Shapira *et al.*, 2005).

Williams syndrome

Williams syndrome (WS) is caused by a deletion of part of chromosome 7. It occurs in one in 20 000 to 30 000 births (Bellugi *et al.*, 1999). Children with Williams syndrome have short stature, wavy hair, hypoplastic teeth, a hoarse voice, blue eyes with a stellate pattern of the iris, and congenital heart disease, usually supravalvular aortic stenosis. As infants, they may have had hypercalcaemia. The cognitive phenotype is characterized by intellectual disability in the upper moderate range on average. Perceptual function is more impaired than verbal and memory function. WS children perform better than mental age-matched controls on all aspects of language phonological, lexical, morphological and syntactic (Bellugi *et al.*, 1999). WS children are able to draw people better than the shapes of other objects (Dykens *et al.*, 2001). A striking feature of Williams syndrome is a characteristic personality style. This is usually called hyper-sociability or indiscriminate sociability. However, WS individuals also have a number of behavioural or emotional problems to a greater extent than IQ-matched controls. They suffer from high levels of anxiety, sleep disturbance and hyperacusis (Einfeld *et al.*, 2001). Specific phobias are more common than generalized anxiety (Dykens, 2003).

Velocardiofacial syndrome

Velocardiofacial syndrome (VCFS) is a consequence of a deletion at 22q11.2. It occurs in about 1 in 3000 live births. Individuals with VCFS often have mild intellectual disability, but may have intelligence in the normal range. As children, they are often shy and withdrawn with a bland affect. In adolescence or young adulthood, psychosis emerges in a high proportion of cases. In a large series, Murphy and colleagues (Murphy *et al.*, 1999b) found a prevalence of psychosis of 30%, the majority of which was schizophrenia.

Down syndrome

Down syndrome is the most common genetic cause of intellectual disability. A number of studies have demonstrated that individuals with Down syndrome have lower levels of behaviour disturbance than others with intellectual disability due to other causes (Tonge and Einfeld, 2003).

Alzheimer-type dementia occurs at an increased rate in Down syndrome and commences at an earlier age. It is also associated with earlier onset of menopause in Down syndrome women (Schupf *et al.*, 2003).

Figure 4.1 shows the level of overall behaviour disturbance in cohorts with these disorders, as measured by the Developmental Behavior Checklist. The epidemiological group derives from a survey of children and adolescents with intellectual disabilities of all causes identified through census regions. The children and adolescents with Williams syndrome and Prader–Willi syndrome have significantly higher rates of disturbance than those with Fragile X or Down syndrome, or those in an epidemiological sample of children with intellectual handicap due to a range of causes (Tonge and Einfeld, 2003).

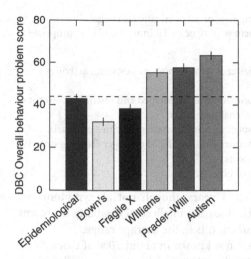

Fig 4.1. Severity of behavioural and emotional disturbance according to syndrome group.

Psychiatric disorders with significant biological origin

Autism spectrum disorders

Autism spectrum disorders are termed in DSM-IV pervasive developmental disorders. They comprise a triad of impairments. The following description is adapted from DSM-IV (American Psychiatric Association, 1994):

Qualitative impairment in social interaction,
    as manifested by:
1. marked impairments in the use of multiple nonverbal behaviors such as eye-to-eye gaze, facial expression, body posture and gestures to regulate social interaction;
2. failure to develop peer relationships appropriate to developmental level;
3. a lack of spontaneous seeking to share enjoyment, interests, or achievements with other people (e.g. by a lack of showing, bringing, or pointing out objects of interest to other people);
4. lack of social or emotional reciprocity (note: in the description, it gives the following as examples: not actively participating in simple social play or games, preferring solitary activities, or involving others in activities only as tools or 'mechanical' aids).

Qualitative impairments in communication
    as manifested by:
1. delay in, or total lack of, the development of spoken language (not accompanied by an attempt to compensate through alternative modes of communication such as gesture or mime);
2. in individuals with adequate speech, marked impairment in the ability to initiate or sustain a conversation with others;

3. stereotyped and repetitive use of language or idiosyncratic language;
4. lack of varied, spontaneous make-believe play or social imitative play appropriate to developmental level.

Restricted repetitive and stereotyped patterns of behavior, interests and activities as manifested by:
1. encompassing preoccupation with one or more stereotyped and restricted patterns of interest that is abnormal either in intensity or focus;
2. apparently inflexible adherence to specific, non-functional routines or rituals;
3. stereotyped and repetitive motor mannerisms (e.g. hand or finger flapping or twisting, or complex whole-body movements);
4. persistent preoccupation with parts of objects.

The symptoms are apparent by age 3 years, though not all symptoms are evident in all individuals. In Autistic disorder, intellectual disability is present. In Asperger disorder, intellectual function is in the average range.

The cause or causes of autism are not known in about 70% of cases. Some individuals have recognized genetic disorders such as tuberous sclerosis or fragile X syndrome, or brain impairments secondary to congenital infections or brain injury. Recently, improved resolution of cytogenetic studies has revealed a range of small chromosome deletions in individuals with autism. Variation in copy number of genes is also thought likely to explain a proportion of autism pathology. For a review of recent developments in the genetics of autism, see Beaudet (2007).

In addition to the defining behaviours described above, or as a consequence of them, a number of behaviours can present problems in individuals with autism. Many of the diagnostic behaviours express a preference for sameness, predictability or preoccupation with limited interests. Disruption of the opportunity for sameness typically generates marked anxiety. The anxiety may present as tantrums, self-injury, or aggression to others or objects. Anti-anxiety medications often raise the threshold before these behaviours occur, making management of the children easier for families.

Brereton et al. (2006) assessed children with intellectual disability with and without autism and found those with autism to have higher levels of a broad range of behavioural disturbances including symptoms of attention-deficit and hyperactivity.

Mood disorders

Depression is characterized by low mood, accompanied by slowing of thinking and difficulty concentrating and sustaining energy. There may be preoccupation with guilt or depressive suicidal ideas. When depression is severe, changes in body function become apparent. There is change of appetite, poor sleep, typically early morning wakening, and physical movement may be slowed. There is little doubt that depressive illness occurs in even severely intellectually disabled individuals and it is likely that this is significantly underdiagnosed. This is not surprising, as the individual has reduced ability to disclose or describe his or her own mood, and the psychiatrist is thereby denied access to the cardinal symptoms of affective illness. However, the abilities both to conceptualize and report mood states vary widely with level of intellectual disability. Mildly intellectually disabled individuals are often able to report mood states clearly. With more severe intellectual disability, diagnosis relies on nonverbal information. It is sometimes possible to elicit from others a history of recent psychomotor retardation, weight loss, diurnal changes in activity and early morning waking. More frequently though, symptoms may be restricted to a sad facial expression, a diminished pleasure in activities, for example, at a living skills programme, and an increased level of agitation or stereotypic behaviour.

In contrast to depression, manic illness tends to be overdiagnosed, as episodic motor overactivity and excitement are common symptoms among people with intellectual disabilities without corroborative evidence of being part of an affective illness. Manic-depressive illness in people with moderate or severe intellectual disability is more likely where there is a well-documented history of changes in affective symptoms of appropriate cyclical periodicity, especially where there is evidence of a depressive phase.

Sometimes, there may be increases in symptoms that are not typical of mood disorders (e.g. self-injury) occurring either in association with the above mood symptoms or alone in individuals with a history of mood disorder. This gives rise to the possibility that these symptoms are an expression of mood disorder in those individuals, generally with more severe intellectual disability.

Psychosis

Psychotic syndromes are defined by the presence of hallucinations, delusions and/or thought disorder. Two psychotic syndromes seen with relative frequency in people with intellectual disability are delirium and schizophrenia. Delirium is a short-lived condition resulting from some intercurrent disturbance of brain function such as fever, or drug intoxication. Schizophrenia is a chronic disorder which is accompanied by a variably progressive decline in adaptive function and motivation. Syndromes clinically indistinguishable from schizophrenia are seen with increased frequency among people with intellectual disability. Given that the underlying organic brain dysfunction is a likely vulnerability or causative factor in presentation, these presentations could more accurately be called organic delusional and/or hallucinatory syndromes. Deb *et al.* (2001) found that 4.4% of adults with mild to moderate intellectual disability had ICD-10 schizophrenia. Despite this, there is evidence that schizophrenia is overdiagnosed in this population (Aman, 1985). This may derive from the misdiagnosis of hallucinations. For example, carers often describe a patient as conducting conversations with absent persons, or admitting to hearing voices of absent persons. However, if the practitioner spends sufficient time questioning and observing the person, they may explain that he or she is remembering conversations or just thinking about them, rather than perceiving them without stimulus. These memories often centre on troubling relationships or events in the individual's life, and the person has no difficulty in distinguishing between the remembered conversations and current reality. Such conversations with absent persons may be a behavioural habit, albeit a socially inappropriate one, but they do not constitute hallucinations.

Similar caution needs to be exercised in the assessment of possible delusions. For example, workshop staff may report that a person is unjustifiably complaining that staff or peers are against him. It should be remembered that people with intellectual disabilities actually do experience a good deal of criticism, devaluation, mockery and rejection so it is not surprising that some individuals develop a sensitivity to communications from others which could be interpreted as critical. A patient, non-threatening interview will often reveal that the individual has not understood what was said by the workshop staff and that the "persecutory" ideas resolve with explanation. Overall, individuals with intellectual disability who are sensitized and sensitive to perceived criticism are much more common than those with true persecutory delusions (Einfeld, 1992).

Where delusions or hallucinations are truly present, the sophistication of their content is reduced (Aman, 1985). That is, an 18-year-old with an IQ of 50 will not, for example, state that spies are reading his mind via the internet. He may, however, believe that the people on the buses that go past his house are trying to harm him.

Anxiety disorders

Anxiety is frequently seen in persons with intellectual disability and when this is of sufficient severity to impair function, a diagnosis of anxiety disorder is justified. Emerson (2003a) found that 8.7% of children with intellectual disability had an anxiety disorder. Anxiety disorders in general carry substantial genetic vulnerability. The full range of anxiety disorders may occur, that is simple phobia, agoraphobia, social anxiety and obsessive-compulsive disorder. Post-Traumatic Stress Disorder is important, especially in adolescents and adults. Many people with intellectual disabilities have experience repeated verbal abuse, devaluation or physical assault. As a consequence, there is an increased level of arousal, mediated through the hypothalamic–pituitary axis, accompanied by disturbances of sleep and alertness. Given cognitive limitations in interpreting potential threats, the individual may overreact through fear and be aggressive.

General health conditions

Pain

Pain is under-recognized in individuals with intellectual disability, as a consequence of their communication difficulties (Symons *et al.*, 2008). Pain regulation may be disturbed in some causes of intellectual disability. In autism there is often insensitivity or hypersensitivity to pain. Individuals with Williams syndrome may be highly sensitive to particular noises, and this may be associated with challenging behaviours. Pain can reduce the level of adaptive functional behaviour (Breau *et al.*, 2007). In one study, self-injurious behaviour was associated with previously undetected painful conditions in 7 of 28 individuals with self-injury. The behaviour decreased in frequency when the pain was relieved (Bosch *et al.*, 1997).

A search for sources of pain should be a component of all assessments for challenging behaviours, especially when the onset is acute. Commonly identified sources include gastrointestinal pain such as dyspepsia from reflux oesophagitis, or constipation, especially with more severe intellectual disability. Middle ear infections are also common.

Guidelines for healthcare of people with intellectual disability have been formulated that will reduce the likelihood that painful conditions underlying challenging behaviours will be undetected. One form of such guidelines is available at: http://www.iassid.org/pdf/healthguidelines.pdf

Epilepsy

Around 20% to 30% of individuals with intellectual disability are reported to suffer from epilepsy (Matthews *et al.*, 2008). A number of psychiatric syndromes are associated with epilepsy, including complex partial seizures, also known as temporal lobe seizures. In this form of epilepsy, consciousness may be retained for routine activities, and there is no tonic or clonic phase. However, cognition and awareness is impaired. Commonly, an aura is experienced as part of the seizure. This may consist of a disturbance of sensation such as flashing lights, or particular smells. Complex partial seizures are sometimes accompanied by aggressive behaviour, if the individual is confronted or approached. It may not be possible to obtain a history of epileptic aura from those with more than mild intellectual disability. Nevertheless, it is usually possible to gather data which help to determine if a temporal lobe seizure is responsible for the behaviour. Carers can usually determine whether there is disorientation and confusion during the aggressive episode or whether, on the other hand, the episode is a well-organized one, occurring in clear consciousness. If the aggressive behaviour is confined to occasions when the patient strikes someone who approaches and tries to restrain them during a period of confusion, this suggests that temporal lobe epilepsy is a possibility. An EEG with nasopharyngeal leads, or sleep deprivation possibly with continuous monitoring, is sometimes necessary to be confident of diagnosis. In practice, it takes a combination of enthusiastic carers, relatively compliant patient and an experienced neurologist to make such investigations a success.

Another syndrome commonly seen in this population, but one which has received little attention in the literature, is that of increasing irritability and aggression often over a period of 2–3 weeks, terminating with a grandmal fit following which the irritability declines. Rarely, such aggression reaches a level of uncontrolled destructive rage, sometimes called epileptic furore. After a variable period, the cycle is repeated. This syndrome can prove challenging to treat, as phenothiazines sometimes reduce the irritability but lower the seizure threshold, while anticonvulsants may have the opposite effects. If this syndrome is suspected, it is helpful to ask carers to keep a diary charting symptoms of irritability, episodes of convulsions and effects of medication changes. The chart will demonstrate whether the temporal relationship of aggression and convulsions conforms to the cyclical syndrome.

Apart from challenging behaviours that may arise from the seizures themselves, epilepsy itself is not associated with increased levels of psychopathology (Lewis *et al.*, 2000; Matthews *et al.*, 2008).

Effects of medications

Many medications can impact on cognition, emotion and behaviour. Indeed, medications used to treat some challenging behaviours may cause other challenging behaviours. Some of the more commonly encountered impacts on behaviour are listed in Table 4.1 below.

Further information on these medications is provided in Chapter 10.

Table 4.1. Possible behavioural side effects of medication

Class of medication	Possible behavioural side effects
Antipsychotics, e.g. olanzapine, risperidone	Increased appetite, lowered seizure threshold, sedation
Serotonin re-uptake inhibitors used for anxiety or depression	Agitation (fluoxetine), sedation (fluvoxamine)
Tricyclics or tetracyclics used for anxiety or depression	Sedation, increased appetite
Stimulants used for attention-deficit hyperactivity, e.g. dexamphetamine, methylphenidate	Headache, decreased appetite, depression

Temperament

The term temperament refers to behavioural characteristics that are apparent in infancy, relatively persistent over time, highly heritable and of genetic origin in the population. One description of these is provided by the EAS Temperament Scale of Buss and Plomin 1984), which identifies temperaments of emotionality, activity and sociability/shyness. Temperament is distinguished from personality, which is regarded as maturing by adulthood and influenced by both genetics and experience.

Gunn *et al.*, 1981) applied Chess and Thomas' Infant Temperament Scales to infants with Down syndrome. Zion and Jenvey (2006) assessed 100 children with intellectual disability due to a range of causes. Both of these studies have found that children with intellectual disability share the same range of constitutional temperamental variation as observed in normally developing children. Thus the role of the child's temperament needs to be considered in understanding the behaviour of the individual.

5

Behavioural models: the functional significance of challenging behaviour

Since the late 1940s psychologists have sought to apply principles derived from learning theory to the understanding (and potential solution) of social problems; including that of challenging behaviours shown by people with intellectual disabilities. These attempts have been accompanied by, and have made a significant contribution to, marked changes in our understanding of the potential of people with severe intellectual disabilities.

Early demonstrations of the power of very simple behavioural methods played an important role in challenging prevailing ideas that people with severe disabilities had little potential for change (Azrin and Foxx, 1971; Bailey and Meyerson, 1969; Lovaas *et al.*, 1965; Tate and Baroff, 1966; Ullman and Krasner, 1965) and the explicit focus of behavioural approaches on the *environmental determinants* of behaviour stood in stark contrast to the prevailing conception that challenging behaviour was the external manifestations of *internal* pathology. The growing influence of behavioural approaches also helped draw attention to the impact of the environment on the behaviour of people with severe disabilities, including the potential damage done by the types of environments provided within institutional settings (Bijou, 1966).

Applied behaviour analysis

Initial successes in the use of behavioural approaches led, in 1968, to the launch of the *Journal of Applied Behaviour Analysis*. In its first issue Baer, Wolf and Risley described the basic nature of applied behaviour analysis as it *ought* to be practised. They suggested, and reiterated 20 years later, that applied behaviour analytic studies should be (Baer *et al.*, 1968, 1987):

- *applied* – in that the behaviours and events studied should be of importance to society;
- *behavioural* – in that studies should be concerned with what people actually do;

Challenging Behaviour, 3rd edn, ed. Eric Emerson and Stewart L. Einfeld. Published by Cambridge University Press. © E. Emerson and S. L. Einfeld 2011.

- *analytic* – in that studies should provide a 'believable demonstration', usually through demonstrating experimental control, that changes in behaviour are linked to the environmental events postulated;
- *technological* – in that the techniques used to change behaviour are identified and described in a manner that allows their replication;
- *conceptually systematic* – in that the procedures used are shown to be related to basic behavioural principles;
- *effective* – in that socially significant changes in behaviour are achieved; and,
- *general* – in that the behavioural change achieved 'proves durable over time ... appears in a wide variety of possible environments or ... spreads to a wide variety of related behaviours'.

Since then, the practice of applied behaviour analysis has steadily advanced both in its traditional areas of application and in many new fields. The application of applied behaviour analysis to the field of severe intellectual disabilities has primarily focussed on two related areas; enhancing people's competence; and reducing challenging behaviours (Cooper *et al.*, 2006; Jones *et al.*, 2001; O'Reilly *et al.*, 2007; Scotti and Meyer, 1999; Sigafoos *et al.*, 2003; Wehmeyer *et al.*, 2002).

In the context of the present book, applied behavioural analysis revolutionized thinking about the causes and management of seriously challenging behaviours (Carr, 1977). The dominant approach within applied behaviour analysis has been to view challenging behaviours as examples of *operant behaviour*. That is, they are seen as forms of behaviour that are shaped and maintained by their environmental consequences. In this sense, challenging behaviours are seen as functional and adaptive. They are behaviours which have been 'selected' or shaped through the person's interaction with their physical and, more importantly, social world. In lay terms they can be thought of as behaviours through which the person exercises control over key aspects of their environment.

The consequences which shape or maintain behaviour are termed reinforcers. Two types of contingent relationship between behaviour and reinforcers are important in establishing and maintaining operant behaviour.

- *Positive reinforcement* refers to an increase in the rate of a behaviour as a result of the contingent *presentation* of a reinforcing stimulus (positive reinforcer). Illustrative examples of positive reinforcement include pressing a light switch to switch on the lights in a room (operant behaviour = pressing switch; positive reinforcer = light going on), smiling and saying hello to a colleague to initiate further conversation (operant behaviour = smiling and saying 'hello'; positive reinforcer = conversation) and requesting a drink when thirsty (operant behaviour = asking for drink; positive reinforcer = being given a drink).
- *Negative reinforcement* refers to an increase in the rate of a behaviour as a result of the contingent *withdrawal* (or prevention of occurrence) of a

reinforcing stimulus (negative reinforcer). Illustrative examples of negative reinforcement include completion of a piece of work to escape from being hassled by your manager (operant behaviour = completion of work; negative reinforcer = withdrawal of/escape from demands) and the *avoidance* of potential crashes and fines by stopping at red traffic lights when driving (operant behaviour = stopping at red lights; negative reinforcer: avoidance of fines and/or crashes).

The operant approach to understanding behaviour has three important characteristics. First, it is concerned with the discovery of *functional relationships* between behaviours and environmental factors. Second, it places a strong emphasis on the importance of the *context* in which behaviour occurs. Finally, it views the behaviours shown by a person as the product of a *dynamic system*.

Functional relationships

Applied behaviour analysis focuses on the discovery of functional relationships between events. This is illustrated in the definitions of reinforcing and punishing stimuli, response classes and in the nature of credible evidence within behaviour analysis. In behavioural theory, reinforcing stimuli are defined functionally. That is, they are defined solely in terms of the impact which their withdrawal or presentation has upon subsequent behaviour. Positive reinforcers, for example, are those stimuli that increase the rate of a behaviour. They cannot be defined or identified independently of their function. That is, no *a priori* assumptions are made regarding whether particular types or classes of stimuli are reinforcing.

The concern within applied behaviour analysis with the analysis of functional relationships also extends to the way in which behaviour is classified. So far, we have used the term operant behaviour. It would be more accurate, however (from the perspective of behavioural theory), to talk about behaviours which are members of an operant *response class*. In a behavioural analysis, attention is normally directed to determining the effect (or function) that a person's behaviour may have upon their environment, not the particular form (or topography) of behaviour. For example, a behaviourist would be interested in understanding the conditions under which you pressed a light switch rather than on how you pressed it (e.g. with your fingers, elbow, arm, nose). Behaviours which result in the same environmental effects are classified as members of the same response class. In most experimental research the focus of attention lies in the environmental determinants or control of response classes. Little attention has been paid to examining the inter-relationships between the actual behaviours which may be members of a particular response class (Mace, 1994).

Finally, the concern of behaviour analysts with the study of functional relationships and their reliance on functional definitions has implications with regard to what is seen as 'credible evidence' in behavioural studies. As we have seen, one implication of defining reinforcement contingencies functionally is that such relationships need to be demonstrated. The notion that credible evidence requires experimental manipulation is reflected in the suggestion that applied behaviour analysis should provide a 'believable demonstration', *through demonstrating experimental control,* that observed changes in behaviour are linked to the suggested environmental events (Baer *et al.,* 1968, 1987). This reliance on the use of experimental control to provide 'believable demonstrations' has (at times quite unhelpfully) focused attention almost exclusively on the relation between challenging behaviour and a very limited range of proximal environmental factors.

Contextual control

Analysis of the context in which behaviour occurs is fundamental to the behaviour analytic perspective. Context influences behaviour in two very different ways. First, it establishes the motivational base that underlies behaviour. Second, it may provide important information or clues to the individual concerning the probability that particular behaviours will be reinforced.

As we have seen, the behavioural approach makes no assumptions regarding whether particular events will function as reinforcers. Instead, behavioural theory suggests that the reinforcing power of stimuli needs to be *established* by contextual relations (Bijou and Baer, 1978; Kantor, 1959; Michael, 1982; Wahler and Fox, 1981). For example, food is only likely to operate as a positive reinforcer if a person is denied free access to it and also if, among other things, they have not recently eaten. Indeed, food could in other contexts (e.g. during food poisoning) operate as a negative reinforcer (increasing behaviours which lead to the withdrawal or postponement of the presentation of food) or a positive punisher (decreasing behaviours which are 'rewarded' by the presentation of food). Similarly, a particular classroom task may only become aversive (and consequently become established as a negative reinforcer) for a child when repeated many times in a short period, when presented in a noisy or stressful setting or when the child is ill. Social contact with adults may become aversive after the experience of sexual abuse. That is, personal, biological, historical and environmental contexts influence the motivational basis of behaviour by determining or establishing the reinforcing and punishing potential of otherwise neutral stimuli. Jack Michael introduced the term *establishing operation* to describe such relationships (Michael, 1982, 1993). He defined this as 'any change in the environment which alters the effectiveness of some object or event as reinforcement and simultaneously alters the momentary frequency of the behaviour that has been followed by that reinforcement'. Since then the notion of establishing operations has undergone significant development (Iwata *et al.,* 2000; Laraway *et al.,* 2003;

McGill, 1999; Michael, 2000). The basic idea, however, remains quite simple and critically important: *historical and current contexts combine to establish the motivational basis of behaviour.*

In addition to this motivational influence, aspects of the contexts in which behaviour occurs may gain 'informational value' through the person's learning history. That is, contextual *discriminative stimuli* distinguish between situations in which specific (reinforcing) consequences for a given behaviour are more or less likely. So, for example, an 'out of order' notice on a lift provides information regarding the operation (or not) of a particular contingency (the probability of button pressing being followed by the appearance of a lift). The difference between these two general classes of antecedent or contextual stimuli is crucial. In lay terms, establishing operations and stimuli change 'people's behaviour by changing what they want ... [as opposed to discriminative or conditional stimuli, which change] ... their chances of getting something that they already want' (Michael, 1982).

These basic arrangements among A(ntecedent):B(ehaviour):C(onsequence) comprise what is commonly described as the *three-term contingency*, which defines *discriminated operant behaviour*, that is operant or 'voluntary' behaviour that shows contextual sensitivity to informational as well as motivational factors.

In recent years, behavioural theory has focused on a related aspect of contextual control: the role of verbal rules in regulating behaviour. This is crucial to our understanding of much human behaviour. While the operant behaviour of non-humans is directly shaped by reinforcement contingencies, much human behaviour is *rule-governed* (Skinner, 1966). That is, it is suggested that verbal rules (instructions and self-instructions) play an important role in mediating and moderating the relationships between actual environmental contingencies and our behaviour.

An example of the importance of verbal rules is provided by the comparison of the performance of people and non-humans on a very simple experimental task. On a fixed-interval schedule of reinforcement, the reinforcer (e.g. food, money, points) becomes available after a *fixed* period of time has elapsed since it was last presented (e.g. 30 seconds). In this situation it does not matter at all what the person does in the intervening period. The most cost-efficient strategy is simply to wait for the fixed period of time to finish, respond in order to access the reinforcer and then wait. Non-humans very rarely do this. Typically, their rate of responding (e.g. lever pressing) will increase in rate during the 'waiting' interval. However, adult humans (who are naïve to the nature of the task) usually do one of two things. Either they show the type of efficient pattern of responding described above (wait – respond – wait – respond), or they show a consistently high rate of responding throughout (a remarkably inefficient strategy). It is likely that the difference is related to the verbal rules people have formulated about the task (Lowe, 1979). People who show the (efficient) low rate of responding tend to describe the nature of the task reasonably accurately (e.g. being able to earn points after waiting for a while). People who show the (inefficient) high rate of responding, however, tend to describe the task (inaccurately) as one in which points are earned on the basis of *how many times* they respond.

While trivial in itself, this example does illustrate two important points. First, verbal rules (or self-instructions) formulated by people about the task (rather than the actual environmental contingencies themselves) appear to determine behaviour. Second, such rules may lead to inefficient (or inaccurate) performance. Indeed, one of the characteristics of rule-governed behaviour is its tendency to make people insensitive to changes in the actual contingencies operating on behaviour (Hayes, 1989).

The key question (given our current interests in understanding the behaviour of people with *severe* intellectual disabilities) is at what stage of verbal development is rule-governed behaviour likely to emerge. Unfortunately, there is no clear answer to this issue. The only safe assumption, it would appear, is that the concept of rule-governed behaviour *may* have some relevance to the explanation of the challenging behaviours shown by people with severe intellectual disabilities. It is, however, highly relevant to understanding the behaviour of carers and staff toward people with challenging behaviour (Hastings and Remington, 1994). This latter point will be discussed in more detail in later chapters.

Behavioural systems

In the real world, we live, work and play in settings in which we could potentially engage in an enormous range of behaviours *all* of which will be under the control of different rules and reinforcement contingencies. As a result, what we actually do needs to be seen as the product of a complex and dynamic behavioural system, rather than reflecting the operation of one discrete contingency on a particular behaviour. The study of variables influencing choice between competing alternative behaviours has been at the forefront of experimental behavioural research for many years (Mace, 1994). We will return to this issue in later chapters.

Applied behaviour analysis and challenging behaviour

Viewing challenging behaviour as an example of operant behaviour opened up two avenues of approach. First, in primarily analytic studies, it led to the search for the contextual factors and environmental consequences responsible for maintaining challenging behaviours. Second, it opened up the possibility of developing approaches to intervention based on either the modification of naturally occurring contingencies or the introduction of new contingencies in order to reduce the rate of the challenging behaviour.

In the following sections we will briefly review evidence that challenging behaviours shown by people with severe intellectual disabilities may be maintained by their environmental consequences. Following this, we will review the evidence supporting a parallel notion, that challenging behaviours may be maintained by their *internal* consequences. Finally, we will briefly mention alternative behavioural approaches to understanding challenging behaviour.

Positive and negative reinforcement

These approaches suggest that challenging behaviour may be maintained by a process of either positive or negative reinforcement. This idea is represented schematically (and simplistically) in Fig. 5.1. First, aspects of the personal and environmental context produce a particular motivational state (and establish the reinforcing potential of events, activities and stimuli). They also, when matched with a particular learning history and the presence of discriminative stimuli which signal the availability of reinforcement, may precipitate an episode of challenging behaviour. Reinforcement of the challenging behaviour will contribute to the person's learning history by increasing the probability

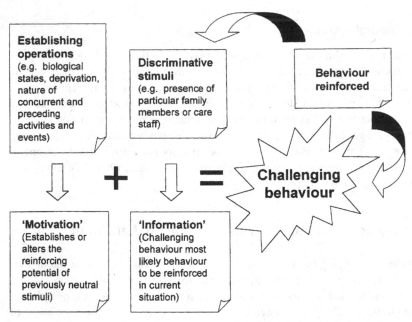

Fig 5.1. Schematic representation of the operant model of challenging behaviour.

that such behaviour is likely to occur in the future in response to similar motivational and environmental conditions.

For example, let us assume that a young man with severe intellectual disabilities has not eaten for a number of hours and is hungry (biological state). Sitting in the lounge of his home with little to do, but with no obvious threats to his immediate safety (environmental context), he would quite like something to eat (motivational state: food becomes established as a potential positive reinforcer). He has neither the skills (personal context: skills) nor opportunity (environmental context) to prepare his own food. A member of his support team wanders in with a burger (environmental context: discriminative stimulus indicating presence of food and presence of someone capable of providing food). As a result of previous learning (personal context: learning history), he begins to bite his hand. The member of staff, who is trying to eat his hamburger, correctly guesses that he is 'communicating' his desire to have something to eat and asks a colleague in the kitchen to bring the young man a biscuit (positive reinforcement: delivery of food).

In another scenario, a young woman with severe intellectual disabilities had a poor night's sleep and is feeling irritable (personal context: biological state). She is asked to complete a difficult task in her noisy and hot supported work placement (environmental context). This combination of factors makes her feel very stressed indeed (motivational state: work tasks become established as a negative reinforcer). She has neither the negotiating skills (personal context: skills) nor opportunity (environmental context) to postpone the task. A sympathetic work colleague comes over (environmental context: discriminative stimuli indicating possibility of escape). As a result of her previous experience (personal context: learning history), she begins to bite her hand. The sympathetic colleague notices her distress, feels upset at the sight of it and persuades her job coach to let her have a break (negative reinforcement: escape from work task).

Each of these examples has three common themes.

- First, a motivational state is established by the interaction of personal (biological) and environmental conditions. This motivational set establishes the reinforcing potential of otherwise neutral stimuli (food; work tasks).
- Second, through previous experience, the person has learned that specific 'challenging' behaviours are more likely to be reinforced by the presentation/ withdrawal of these reinforcers under certain conditions (particular discriminative stimuli in the form of members of staff or co-workers).
- Finally, the *co-occurrence* of the motivation state and discriminative stimuli evokes an episode of challenging behaviour which is subsequently reinforced by contingent presentation (or withdrawal) of the pertinent reinforcer.

Four sources of evidence indicate that some examples of challenging behaviours shown by people with severe intellectual disabilities may be maintained by their environmental consequences.

Descriptive studies

At the simplest level, a number of descriptive studies have examined aspects of the social context in which challenging behaviours occur. Edelson and colleagues, for example, observed 20 young people with intellectual disabilities residing in a state institution in North America (Edelson *et al.*, 1983). They recorded occurrences of self-injurious behaviour and various staff behaviours directed towards the young person (e.g. demands, denial, punishment, praise), finding that, for 19/20 participants, rates of self-injury increased significantly immediately following staff demands, denials or punishment. Whilst other explanations cannot be ruled out, such results are consistent with the notion that the participants' self-injury may have been maintained by a process of negative reinforcement. That is, the presentation of a potential negative reinforcer (staff contact) may have elicited the behaviour (self-injury) which may have been reinforced in the past by the subsequent withdrawal of staff contact. Since then, studies have used increasingly sophisticated observational techniques to document the extent to which challenging behaviours are systematically related to key aspects of the person's immediate social environment (Borrero and Borrero, 2008; Camp *et al.*, 2009; Emerson *et al.*, 1995; Emerson *et al.*, 1996b; Hall and Oliver, 2000; Martens *et al.*, 2008; McComas *et al.*, 2009; Pence *et al.*, 2009; Samaha *et al.*, 2009; Toogood and Timlin, 1996).

Experimental demonstrations of the contextual control of challenging behaviour

Perhaps more convincing evidence is provided by *experimental demonstration* of the contextual control of challenging behaviour. Brian Iwata and colleagues, in a seminal study, examined the effect of context on the self-injurious behaviour of nine children with intellectual disabilities (Iwata *et al.*, 1982). They recorded the rates of self-injury shown under four different experimental conditions. In the *social disapproval* condition an adult was present throughout, but did not interact with the child except to express concern or mild disapproval (e.g. 'don't do that') on the occurrence of self-injury. This condition was assumed to be discriminative for the occurrence of self-injury maintained by positive social reinforcement. In the *academic demand* condition an adult was present throughout and encouraged the child to complete an educational task using a graduated (ask–show–guide) prompting procedure. However, the adult withdrew their attention contingent on self-injury shown by the child. Such a condition was assumed to be discriminative for self-injury maintained by negative social reinforcement (i.e. escape from demands). In the *alone* condition no adults or materials were present. Such a condition was assumed to be discriminative for behaviours maintained by automatic or perceptual reinforcement (see below). The *control* condition consisted of a stimulating environment in which social attention is delivered contingent upon the non-occurrence of self-injury. One-third of the children showed patterns of self-injury that were consistent with their behaviour being maintained by environmental consequences.

Since then, Iwata's research group have summarized the results of such *experimental functional analyses* for 152 people with intellectual disabilities who showed self-injurious behaviour (Iwata *et al.*, 1994b). Of these, 93% (142) had a severe intellectual disability. Of the 152 people: 38% showed patterns of responding consistent with their self-injury being maintained by negative reinforcement; 26% showed patterns of responding consistent with their self-injury being maintained by positive reinforcement; 21% showed patterns of responding consistent with their self-injury being maintained by internal or automatic reinforcement; 5% showed patterns of responding consistent with their self-injury being maintained by multiple controlling variables (e.g. positive and negative reinforcement); 10% showed undifferentiated or unpredictable patterns of responding.

Similar medium-scale studies have suggested that:
- 29% of various forms of challenging behaviour shown by 79 people with intellectual disabilities were maintained by negative reinforcement, 22% by positive reinforcement and 15% by automatic reinforcement (the remaining 34% were unclear) (Derby *et al.*, 1992);
- 46% of various forms of challenging behaviour shown by 28 young children with developmental disabilities were maintained by negative reinforcement, 21% by positive reinforcement, 18% by positive and negative reinforcement and 4% by automatic reinforcement (the remaining 11% were unclear) (Wacker *et al.*, 1998);
- 3% of various forms of self-injury shown by 29 children with intellectual disabilities were maintained by negative reinforcement, 38% by positive reinforcement, 7% by positive and negative reinforcement, and 14% by automatic reinforcement (the remaining 38% were unclear) (Kurtz *et al.*, 2003);
- 39% of various forms of challenging behaviour shown by 119 people with developmental disabilities were maintained by positive and negative reinforcement, 27% by negative reinforcement, 14% by positive reinforcement, 9% by automatic reinforcement and one or more forms of social reinforcement and 7% by automatic reinforcement (the remaining 4% were unclear) (Asmus *et al.*, 2004).

Combining results across these four studies suggests that the majority (71%) of challenging behaviours assessed appeared to be maintained by some form of some form of social (positive or negative) reinforcement and that negative reinforcement (escape) was more common than positive reinforcement (attention) (46% vs. 37%). In behaviour analytic terms these experimental functional analyses have provided 'believable demonstrations', for many participants, of a form of contextual control over challenging behaviour which is consistent with the operant (positive/negative reinforcement) hypothesis (Hanley *et al.*, 2003).

A growing number of studies have taken this issue further by demonstrating the contextual control of the types of (apparently) functional relationships. That is, they have provided data that are consistent with the role played by contextual *establishing operations* in creating the conditions under which processes of positive or negative reinforcement may or may not occur. In one of the earliest of such studies, Carr and colleagues demonstrated that the self-injurious head hitting shown by Tim, an 8-year-old boy with intellectual disabilities and autism, was reliably elicited by adult requests (compared with other types of interaction and free time) (Carr *et al.*, 1976). They then went on to show that *changing the context* in which the requests were made brought about dramatic changes in Tim's behaviour. When interaction consisted solely of making requests his self-injury occurred, as previously, at very high rates. However, when the time between making the same requests was filled with telling Tim a story, his self-injury immediately dropped to near zero levels. Perhaps the most plausible explanation of these results is that adult requests functioned, in certain contexts, as a negative reinforcer for Tim's self-injury (i.e. he had in the past learned that his self-injury would lead to the withdrawal of requests). What is particularly interesting in this study, however, is the dramatic demonstration of the contextual control of this functional relationship. Relatively small changes in the situation (telling a story) appeared to be capable of totally disrupting this powerful relationship.

More recent studies have identified a wide range of variables which, for particular individuals, appear to determine whether challenging behaviours are likely to occur under the types of environmental conditions that are consistent with the behaviour being maintained by a process of positive or negative reinforcement. These have included illness or pain, sleep deprivation, food deprivation, mood, location, prior activity, concurrent activities, the presence of such idiosyncratic variables such as small balls, puzzles and magazines (Carr and Smith, 1995; Carr *et al.*, 1996; Carr *et al.*, 1997; Kennedy and Meyer, 1998; Kennedy and Becker, 2006; Kern *et al.*, 2006; Kuhn *et al.*, 2009; Lang *et al.*, 2008; Lang *et al.*, 2009a).

Experimental manipulations of the reinforcing contingencies hypothesized to be maintaining challenging behaviour

The strongest evidence in support of the operant model is provided by those studies that have demonstrated control over challenging behaviours by manipulating the contingencies of reinforcement which are hypothesized to maintain them. If a behaviour is maintained by a process of positive reinforcement, preventing the reinforcer occurring contingent on the behaviour should lead to the *extinction* of the behaviour. Similarly, if a behaviour is maintained by a process of negative reinforcement, preventing the withdrawal of the reinforcer contingent on the behaviour should lead to the extinction of the behaviour. (The latter technique is referred to as negative or escape extinction.)

Some of the earliest evidence supporting the operant model used this approach (Lerman and Iwata, 1996). Lovaas and Simmons, for example, demonstrated that withholding adult attention led to the extinction of the severe self-injurious behaviours shown by two boys with severe intellectual disabilities (Lovaas and Simmons, 1969). They then went on to re-instate, before finally eliminating, the self-injury shown by one of the boys by providing 'comforting' attention contingent on his self-injury. The 'comforting' attention that led to a rapid *worsening* of his self-injury consisted of such natural responses as holding his hand and re-assuring him that everything was 'OK'. Lovaas has subsequently referred to such 'humane' reactions as an example of 'benevolent enslavement', in that the good intentions of carers in comforting the child appeared themselves primarily responsible for maintaining the self-injury (Lovaas, 1982).

Experimental manipulations of the reinforcing contingencies hypothesized to be maintaining other behaviours belonging to the same response class as the person's challenging behaviour

Finally, a number of studies have provided strong evidence in support of the operant model by demonstrating functional control over challenging behaviour by *differentially reinforcing* a more socially appropriate member of the same response class. That is, they have identified the behavioural function of the person's challenging behaviour (e.g. to escape from teacher demands, to elicit teacher attention). They have then taught and systematically reinforced a *functionally equivalent* response (e.g. to request a break as an alternative to escape motivated challenging behaviour). Under conditions which are themselves predictable from behavioural theory, this approach can lead to rapid and significant reductions in the person's challenging behaviour (Carr and Durand, 1985a; Durand et al., 1993).

These studies, in combination, provide strong evidence to support the proposition that some examples of challenging behaviours shown by people with severe intellectual disabilities may be maintained by processes of either positive or negative reinforcement.

All the examples of negative reinforcement that have been discussed have involved the person's challenging behaviour acting as an *escape* behaviour (i.e. leading to escape from, or withdrawal of, the negative reinforcer). Given that this appears to be the most prevalent behavioural function, it is probable that some examples of challenging behaviours may also function as *avoidance* behaviours. That is, they may serve to prevent, postpone or delay the presentation of (aversive) negative reinforcers. For example, carers may have learned to avoid presenting negative reinforcers (e.g. social demands) under conditions in which the person with intellectual disabilities appears distressed (e.g. by exhibiting low level repetitive self-injurious behaviour). In such a situation, self-injurious behaviour would serve to avoid (postpone or prevent) the occurrence of demands.

If this were the case, then we would expect (assuming the avoidance behaviour was under some form of discriminative control) that the behaviour would occur under conditions in which the negative reinforcer (demands) was more likely to occur. If it operated as a *successful* avoidance behaviour, however, we would not see *any* environmental consequences of the behaviour as the maintaining contingency involves the non-occurrence of a potential event (the negative reinforcer). To an observer, therefore, the person's challenging behaviour would appear to have no consequence and, unless very precise discriminative control had been established, to have no clear antecedents. Nevertheless, it would still be an example of operant behaviour maintained by its environmental consequences.

Processes of negative reinforcement can also be used to account for the process of 'benevolent enslavement' (Carr *et al.*, 1991; Oliver, 1993; Taylor and Carr, 1993). In both of the hypothetical examples with which we started this section, the cessation of an individual's challenging behaviour may be thought of as negatively reinforcing the action of care staff. In these examples, the person's challenging behaviour may act as a negative reinforcer which is withdrawn contingent upon the 'helping' behaviours of care staff (providing food, withdrawing demands). The staff behaviour which reinforces the person's challenging behaviour is itself reinforced by the termination of the challenging behaviour. Thus, carer and user get locked in a viscous circle (or negative reinforcement trap) which perpetuates the person's challenging behaviour.

If this is the case, then we may expect two further things to happen. First, carers and care staff are likely to habituate (get used to) particular intensities or forms of challenging behaviour over time. Thus, they may begin to only respond (and hence provide contingent reinforcement) when the person shows *more intense* or *more complex* forms of challenging behaviour. This is, of course, the basis of all shaping procedures in which new behaviours are taught by differentially reinforcing particular aspects of the behaviour which the person already shows. In this case, however, the possibility of carers and care staff habituating to 'ordinary' levels of challenging behaviour may lead to the systematic (but unplanned) shaping of more and more intense or complex forms of the behaviour. Such a process may partially account for the development of challenging behaviour (Guess and Carr, 1991; Oliver, 1993).

In addition, if the termination of challenging behaviour acts as a negative reinforcer, we may also expect carers and care staff to develop strategies for *avoiding* the occurrence of such behaviours. So, people may come to avoid interacting with users whose challenging behaviours are maintained by processes of negative social reinforcement (e.g. escape from demands, escape from social attention), while increasing their rates of interaction with users whose challenging behaviour is maintained by processes of positive social reinforcement (e.g. access to social attention). Taylor and her colleagues have demonstrated that such a pattern is quite rapidly established and is sufficiently robust to be used to predict the functions served by challenging behaviours (Carr et al., 1991; Taylor and Carr, 1993).

Automatic reinforcement

It is clear that not all behaviour is shaped by its environmental consequences. Some behaviours are innate (e.g. salivating at the sight of food when hungry). Others are learned reflexive behaviours that are elicited by environmental stimuli (e.g. salivating at the sound of a dinner bell when hungry). Others appear to be maintained by consequences internal to the person (e.g. clenching your teeth may attenuate the pain from a sprained ankle, scratching an insect bite may temporarily relieve the sensation of itching).

It has been suggested that this latter class of behaviours may be thought of as examples of operant behaviour maintained by a process of automatic or perceptual reinforcement, in which the reinforcing stimuli are private or internal to the person (Berkson, 1983; Carr, 1977; Lovaas et al., 1987; Vollmer, 1994). Potential internal or automatic reinforcers include perceptual feedback from the response itself (e.g. visual effects of eye poking, kinaesthetic feedback from rocking, visual and auditory feedback from spinning toys), modulation of levels of arousal, relief from itching and the attenuation of pain.

While this approach is not without its problems for behaviour analysts (Kennedy, 1994b), circumstantial support for the notion of automatic or perceptual reinforcement is provided by a number of studies. First, studies have indicated that the probability of occurrence of some forms of challenging behaviour (primarily stereotypy and self-injury) varies with the level of general environmental stimulation. As has been discussed above, a significant proportion of challenging behaviours occur at their highest rates under conditions of social and material deprivation. Similarly, a number of studies have shown that increasing the level of environmental stimulation may lead to reductions in stereotypic and other forms of challenging behaviour (Favell et al., 1982; Horner, 1980).

Interestingly, however, exactly the opposite results have been obtained in other studies. Duker and Rasing (1989), for example, found that *decreasing* the level of stimulation in the classroom by removing furniture, pictures and extraneous materials led to a reduction in stereotyped behaviour (and increase in on-task behaviour) among young adults with autism (Duker and Rasing, 1989). These results are consistent with an alternative explanation; that some forms of challenging behaviour may be maintained by a process of negative automatic reinforcement in that they serve to actively dampen (aversive) levels of overarousal.

Further circumstantial evidence for the operation of automatic reinforcement is provided by the impact of *sensory extinction* in reducing some forms of challenging behaviour, a procedure that involves masking the sensory consequences arising from the behaviour (Rincover and Devany, 1982). Of course, none of this evidence is particularly convincing, due to the inability or failure to independently measure the hypothesized internal consequences of the challenging behaviour.

Other behavioural processes

Respondent behaviour

Respondent behaviours are those reflexive or conditioned behaviours which are primarily involuntary in nature (e.g. blinking, salivating, changes in heart rate, skin conductance). While a considerable amount of behavioural theorizing about issues of arousal and anxiety in non-disabled people has viewed them as examples of acquired or conditioned respondent behaviours (e.g. phobic fear), there has been remarkably little attention paid to issues of anxiety and arousal among people with severe intellectual disabilities (Romanczyk et al., 1992; Romanczyk and Matthews, 1998). It has been suggested that anxiety and arousal may play some role in the maintenance of self-injurious behaviour, in that: (1) self-injury may be elicited as a reflexive response to high levels of arousal generated by environmental stressors; (2) self-injury can itself generate high levels of arousal. Similarly, evidence from basic research has indicated that aggression may be elicited as a reflexive response by punishment (Hutchinson, 1977).

Schedule induced behaviour

Under conditions involving the repetitive delivery of food on a fixed-time schedule, or under some examples of fixed-interval schedules of reinforcement, schedule-induced behaviours may appear. These are behaviours which occur in the period immediately following reinforcement, are excessive, stereotyped in appearance, unrelated to the demands of the situation and often highly persistent over time (Staddon, 1977). While the majority of studies of schedule induced behaviour have taken place in the animal laboratory, a few studies have suggested the process may have some relevance to the understanding of stereotypic behaviour in people with intellectual disabilities (Emerson and Howard, 1992; Emerson et al., 1996c; Lerman et al., 1994).

Summary

The studies which have been reviewed in this chapter provide strong evidence that many examples of challenging behaviours shown by people with severe intellectual disabilities are maintained by behavioural processes. The operant model also provides a coherent account of the types of reciprocal influences between people with intellectual disabilities and carers which may lead to the development of challenging behaviour (Guess and Carr, 1991; Oliver, 1993) and its maintenance through the process of 'benevolent enslavement' (Taylor and Carr, 1993).

Romanczyk and his colleagues, however, warn us that to label challenging behaviour as adaptive and functional 'provides a perspective superior to viewing it simply as a psychotic behaviour but also lends itself to a simplistic and naive understanding as well ... one cannot assume that the causal and maintaining factors are (1) similar across individuals, (2) consistent for the same individual at different points in time, and (3) similar for different topographies of [challenging] ... behaviour both within and across individuals' (Romanczyk et al., 1992). To this, it could be added that we cannot assume that causal and maintaining factors are (4) consistent for the same individual across different contexts and (5) not complex and diverse within specific topographies. Indeed, the variety of possible behavioural functions and aetiological processes, the frequent co-occurrence of different forms of challenging behaviours and the importance of the contextual control of behavioural relationships should all serve to guard us against such naivety.

6

Broader environmental influences on challenging behaviour

The two great strengths of behavioural approaches were, first and foremost, to draw attention to potential environmental determinants of challenging behaviour and, second, to adopt a stringent approach to evidence that established without doubt that *for some people* environmental determinants are central to understanding their challenging behaviour. Within these strengths, however, also lie the roots of some of the weaknesses of behavioural perspectives. In particular, the particular approach to evidence adopted within the applied behavioural research community (presenting a 'believable demonstration' through establishing *experimental* control), when combined with the potential powerful effects of altering reinforcement contingencies, has focused attention almost exclusively on the role of proximal environmental determinants of challenging behaviour that can be readily manipulated and brought under experimental control. While the potential limitations and narrowness of such an approach have long been recognized (Morris and Midgley, 1990; Willems, 1974), such concerns have had relatively little impact on applied behavioural research.

In this chapter we will review the evidence that suggests that understanding and effectively responding to the challenging behaviour shown by people with severe intellectual disabilities requires that we take a much broader view of potential environmental influences. But first, a word of warning; little of the evidence we call on in this chapter is specific to challenging behaviour shown by people with severe, rather than mild, intellectual disabilities. The reason for this is quite simple, research on challenging behaviour shown by people with severe intellectual disabilities has been almost completely dominated by either biological or behavioural models, neither of which – in practice – pay more than lip service to the potential importance of the wider environment (one of the reasons why this chapter did not appear in previous versions of this book). We will, however, be drawing on evidence from two related areas: (1) research on 'challenging behaviour' (e.g. violence and aggression) shown by people without intellectual disabilities; and (2) research on behavioural difficulties

Challenging Behaviour, 3rd edn, ed. Eric Emerson and Stewart L. Einfeld. Published by Cambridge University Press. © E. Emerson and S. L. Einfeld 2011.

shown by children with the full range of intellectual disabilities (mild, moderate and severe).

One of the main characteristics of the dominant paradigms in the area of challenging behaviour is the search for ever more proximal or immediate causes of (or mediating pathways to) human functioning. The belief is that the closer and closer we can get to understanding the immediate causes of a phenomenon, the more credible our explanations and the greater our chances of designing effective interventions or supports. Of course, the identification of mediating pathways and immediate (or proximal) causes is critically important in developing a more nuanced understanding of any phenomena and does, of course, open up the possibility of designing 'downstream' interventions that address these immediate (or proximal) causes to address social problems.

It is an error, however, to consider that evidence of mediation reduces the scientific significance or social importance of background (or distal) variables. Indeed, a radically different view is often taken in public health research where the research agenda often focuses explicitly on identifying the distal causes of more proximal events, or, in the words of Professor Sir Michael Marmot (Chair of the World Health Organization Special Commission on the Social Determinants of Health) 'the causes of the causes' (World Health Organization, 2007b, 2008c). Such an approach opens up the possibility of developing 'upstream' interventions that address background (or distal) variables and may have a broad and pervasive impact on health and well-being.

Socio-economic position, poverty and behavioural difficulties

All societies are hierarchically structured, and in all societies a person's position in the social hierarchy will shape their (and their children's) access to, and control over, key resources that play an important role in determining health and well-being (Graham, 2007; World Health Organization, 2008c). People occupying lower socio-economic positions may have difficulty accessing resources that are necessary to enable them to live lives that are considered appropriate or decent within their society. That is, they may experience *poverty* in that they may be unable '*due to lack of resources*, to participate in society and to enjoy a standard of living consistent with human dignity and social decency' (Fabian Commission on Life Chances and Child Poverty, 2006).

Socio-economic position, poverty and the prevalence of intellectual and developmental disability

Although families supporting a person with intellectual or developmental disabilities are located at all points across the social hierarchy, they are – in general – significantly more likely than other families to be located in lower socio-economic positions and to experience poverty (Chapman *et al.*, 2008; Durkin, 2002; Emerson, 2004, 2007; Emerson *et al.*, 2009; Fujiura, 1998; Heber, 1970; Heikura *et al.*, 2008; Leonard and Wen, 2002; Murphy *et al.*, 1988; Parish *et al.*, 2008; Roeleveld *et al.*, 1997). However, the strength of association between socio-economic position and intellectual and developmental disabilities varies significantly by type and severity of disability, with stronger associations being found as the severity of intellectual disability decreases, and little or no association between socio-economic position and the prevalence of autistic spectrum disorder or profound multiple intellectual disability (Baird *et al.*, 2006; Chapman *et al.*, 2008; Emerson *et al.*, 2009). Thus, for some children with intellectual or developmental disabilities (e.g. autistic spectrum disorders, profound multiple intellectual disability) rates of exposure to low socio-economic position or poverty will be similar to that in the wider population. For others, including children with more severe intellectual disabilities, rates of exposure will be somewhat greater than in the wider population.

The impact of socio-economic position on behavioural health and well-being

There now exists a wealth of evidence documenting (in the general population) the negative impact of exposure to low socio-economic position and/or poverty on general behavioural health and well-being (Bornstein and Bradley, 2003; Bradley and Corwyn, 2002; Bradshaw, 2001; Brooks-Gunn and Duncan, 1997; Duncan and Brooks-Gunn, 2000; Graham, 2007; Lister, 2004; Marmot and Wilkinson, 2006; Wilkinson and Pickett, 2009; World Health Organization, 2008). There is also considerable evidence to suggest that exposure to low socio-economic position and/or poverty (and factors associated with low socio-economic position and/or poverty) are strongly related to both the development and persistence of aggression and other behavioural difficulties in children (Broidy *et al.*, 2003; Jenkins, 2008; Maughan *et al.*, 2004; Tremblay, 2000; Tremblay *et al.*, 2004; Tremblay, 2006). Three important themes emerge from this disparate and voluminous literature. Specifically, the negative outcomes associated with low socio-economic position or poverty:

- are related to the duration and depth of exposure (Ackerman *et al.*, 2004; Jarjoura *et al.*, 2002; Lynch *et al.*, 1997; McLeod and Shanahan, 1996; Petterson and Albers, 2004);
- are mediated through a multiplicity of pathways including, but not limited to, increased risk of exposure to a range of material and psychosocial hazards such as exposure to a range of toxins and teratogens, poorer educational and occupational opportunities, adverse life events, poorer health and welfare services, and poorer quality neighbourhoods (Aber *et al.*, 1997; Bradley *et al.*, 2001; Dixon *et al.*, 2008; Evans and Kantrowitz, 2002; Kawachi and Berkman, 2003; Unwin and Deb, 2008). Many of these pathways, however,

are rooted in family functioning and parenting practices (Bradley and Corwyn, 2002; Conger and Conger, 2002; Conger and Donnellan, 2007; Linver *et al.*, 2002);
- may be moderated by a range of factors. Some children and their families are more resilient than others.

There exists a wide-ranging and extensive literature on the issues of vulnerability and resilience in the face of adversity (Coleman and Hagell, 2007; Grant *et al.*, 2006; Haskett *et al.*, 2006; Luthar, 2003, 2006; Luthar and Brown, 2007; Rutter, 1985, 2000; Sandberg and Rutter, 2008; Schoon, 2006; Werner and Smith, 1992). A key message from this literature is that resilient functioning in children and young people is likely to reflect the complex interplay between individual characteristics and attributes (e.g. temperament, intelligence, personality, coping style, religiosity), the relationships with, and characteristics of, their families (e.g. supportive parenting style, family cohesion) and their relationships with, and characteristics of, the wider social context in which they are living (e.g. sense of belongingness to the local community, quality of educational and leisure services, neighbourhood safety). Many of the factors associated with resilient functioning are also related to socio-economic position and/or poverty. As a result, the impact of low socio-economic position/poverty on well-being is likely to operate through both increasing the cumulative risk of exposure to a variety of material and psychosocial hazards *and* by undermining the resilience of the person exposed.

The impact of socio-economic position on the behavioural health and well-being of people with intellectual or developmental disabilities

In the preceding sections we have summarized evidence indicating that: (1) exposure to low socio-economic position and/or poverty has a pervasive detrimental impact on behavioural health and well-being; (2) people with intellectual disabilities are more likely than their non-disabled peers to be exposed to low socio-economic position and/or poverty. Unless people with intellectual disabilities are somehow immune to the types of process that link socio-economic position/poverty to health and well-being in the general population, we should therefore expect exposure to low socio-economic position/poverty to be at least as important in understanding the well-being of people with intellectual disabilities as it is for understanding well-being of other people. There is, unsurprisingly, little or no evidence to suggest that such immunity exists (Emerson and Hatton, 2007d, 2010). For example, we have recently demonstrated that the form of the relationship between breadth of exposure to socio-economic risk and the prevalence of diagnosable conduct disorders is very similar for children with and without intellectual disabilities (Emerson and Hatton, 2007d).

Given that exposure to low socio-economic position and/or poverty has a pervasive detrimental impact on well-being, *and* that people with intellectual disabilities are more likely to be exposed to such circumstances, it seems plausible to suggest that the poorer emotional and behavioural well-being of people with intellectual disabilities may – in part – be attributable to their poorer socio-economic position. Indeed, our recent research suggests that increased exposure to low socio-economic position/poverty may account for: (1) 20%–50% of the increased risk for poorer health and mental health among two nationally representative cohorts of British children and adolescents with intellectual disabilities (Emerson and Hatton, 2007a, 2007b, 2007d); (2) 29%–43% of the increased risk for conduct difficulties and 36%–43% of the increased risk for peer problems among a nationally representative cohort of 6–7-year-old Australian children with intellectual disabilities or borderline intellectual functioning (Emerson *et al.*, 2010); (3) a significant proportion of increased rates of self-reported antisocial behaviour among adolescents with intellectual disability (Dickinson *et al.*, 2007); and (4) 32% of the increased risk for conduct difficulties and 27% of the increased risk for peer problems among a nationally representative cohort of 3-year-old British children with developmental delay (Emerson and Einfeld, 2010). These results also provide evidence that exposure to poverty or low socio-economic position accounts for part of the variation in well-being *among* people with intellectual disabilities (Emerson, 2003c; Emerson *et al.*, 2005, 2007b; Emerson and Hatton, 2007d, 2008a, 2008b; Koskentausta *et al.*, 2006).

As noted above, however, the effects of low socio-economic position or poverty on the well-being of people with intellectual disabilities are likely to be mediated through a number of distinct pathways that are themselves linked to (but not unique to) low socio-economic position. Current evidence suggests that challenging behaviour or mental health problems in people with intellectual disabilities may be associated with the following potential mediating pathways:

- cumulative exposure to acute life stresses or adverse 'life events' (Coe *et al.*, 1999; Cooper *et al.*, 2007; Esbensen and Benson, 2006; Hamilton *et al.*, 2005; Hastings *et al.*, 2004; Hatton and Emerson, 2004; Hulbert-Williams and Hastings, 2008; Monaghan and Soni, 1992; Owen *et al.*, 2004)
- exposure to specific life events such as abuse (Beail and Warden, 1995; Murphy *et al.*, 2007; Sequeira *et al.*, 2003), parental death (Bonell-Pascual *et al.*, 1999; Esbensen *et al.*, 2008) and placement outside the home (Esbensen *et al.*, 2008)
- poorer family functioning (Chadwick *et al.*, 2008; Emerson, 2003c; Hardan and Sahl, 1997; Wallander *et al.*, 2006) and
- being brought up by a single parent (Dekker and Koot, 2003; Emerson, 2003b; Hardan and Sahl, 1997; Koskentausta *et al.*, 2006).

It needs to be kept in mind that exposure to all of these events or situations is significantly more likely among people in lower socio-economic positions. It also needs to be kept in mind that the strength of the evidence of the association between these broader environmental conditions and behavioural difficulties or challenging behaviours is rather weak. Most studies are correlational, most have failed to adequately address the relationships between 'upstream' and (mediating) 'downstream' factors, and most are not specific to people with *severe* intellectual disabilities.

Nevertheless, when taken in the context of the much more robust evidence relating to 'challenging behaviours' shown by people who do not have intellectual disabilities the available evidence suggests this is an area worthy of more detailed study. For example, we are currently in the process of investigating factors associated with the persistence and emergence of behavioural difficulties over a 2-year period in a nationally representative cohort of Australian children with intellectual disabilities or borderline intellectual functioning (Emerson *et al.*, in preparation). Our preliminary results suggest that the *persistence* of severe behavioural difficulties between the ages of 4/5 and 6/7 is two to three times higher among children who experience material hardship, children of single mothers and children whose mothers have mental health problems. However, the *emergence* of severe behavioural difficulties between the ages of 4/5 and 6/7 appears to be related to different aspects of the broader environment, with risk of emergence being over four times greater among children living in deprived communities.

Socio-economic position and intervention

Before leaving this area, it is also worth noting that, whatever the role of the broader social environment in the emergence and persistence of challenging behaviour, understanding the impact of low socio-economic position and poverty on family functioning and personal well-being is likely to be important when designing and implementing interventions and supports. As we have seen, people with intellectual disabilities in general are more likely to be exposed to low socio-economic position and/or poverty and, given the association between low socio-economic position and/or poverty and behavioural difficulties, this will be particularly the case among people with intellectual disabilities who also have behavioural difficulties or challenging behaviour. For example, we have estimated that 57% of all British children who have an intellectual disability and a diagnosable conduct disorder live in poverty (Emerson and Hatton, 2007c).

This simple observation is important on two counts. First, it suggests that the need for support and interventions is going to be significantly higher in more disadvantaged communities. Second, it suggests that any intervention must be fit for purpose and as effective when implemented in more disadvantaged communities as they may be in more advantaged communities. Otherwise, our interventions run the risk of *increasing* social inequality through failing to reach or support the most disadvantaged. This is more than idle speculation, as there exists a very long history of health related interventions that are based on behaviour change being more effective among more advantaged sections of the community (White *et al.*, 2009). These include group based behavioural parent training programmes for parents in general (Lundahl *et al.*, 2006) and among parents of children with intellectual or developmental disabilities (Harris *et al.*, 1991).

7

Making connections

In the last three chapters we have looked at biological, behavioural and broader environmental influences on challenging behaviour. In this chapter we will look at possible connections and overlaps among these three very general perspectives. We are not, however, going to present some grandiose overarching model of challenging behaviour. The main reason for this is that we believe it impossible that any *single* model could cover the multiplicity of independent (and partially independent) pathways that may lead to challenging behaviour. Instead, it is much more likely that our growing understanding of challenging behaviour will reflect the principle of equifinality (i.e. that in 'open' systems, which continuously interact with the environment, a given end state can be reached by many potential means).

What we will attempt to do in this chapter is to examine some of the possible ways in which biological, behavioural and broader environmental factors may interact to either increase or decrease the chances that a person with severe intellectual disabilities may show challenging behaviour. We will focus on two specific areas (biological influences on behavioural processes; and the association between social contexts, parenting and behavioural processes) before addressing the possible biological, behavioural and contextual influences on the development and persistence of challenging behaviour in childhood.

Biological influences as establishing operations in behavioural processes

As we discussed in Chapter 5, behavioural theory suggests that no events or stimuli are intrinsically reinforcing. Rather, the reinforcing properties of events or stimuli result from the influence of establishing operations associated with historical and/or contextual factors. Biological states are likely to constitute a particularly relevant class of establishing operations. Take, for example, the

Challenging Behaviour, 3rd edn, ed. Eric Emerson and Stewart L. Einfeld. Published by Cambridge University Press. © E. Emerson and S. L. Einfeld 2011.

possible associations between pain and challenging behaviour. First, pain (as an aversive stimulus) may directly evoke an episode of 'reflexive' non-functional challenging behaviour (Hutchinson, 1977). Second, some forms of challenging behaviour (e.g. hitting your fist on a table top) may serve to reduce the experience of pain (in which case the challenging behaviour is being negatively reinforced by the reduction in an unobservable internal state through a process of 'automatic reinforcement'). Finally, and perhaps most importantly, pain may have a pervasive effect on establishing the positive and negative reinforcing potential of a wide range of activities and events. When we are in pain, nurturing social contact may become more reinforcing and difficult tasks more aversive. In this scenario, the association between pain and challenging behaviour is indirect. Pain does not cause challenging behaviour, but it does change people's motivational states and may help create the conditions under which challenging behaviour is expressed *if* challenging behaviour has already been established as a functional response in relation to these motivational states (e.g. as an effective means of accessing nurturing social contact, as an effective means of escaping from or avoiding difficult tasks). This is more than just semantics for, as we shall see, this type of association opens up two alternative approaches to intervention including: (1) change the person's motivational state (e.g. by reducing pain); (2) change the functionality of challenging behaviour when that motivational state is present (e.g. by providing a more efficient way for the person to access nurturing social contact or avoid/escape from difficult tasks).

Biological events or states that may act as establishing operations include:

- illness or pain including pain associated with gastroesophageal reflux, otitis media and constipation (Bosch *et al.*, 1997; Carr and Smith, 1995; Carr *et al.*, 1996; Gardner and Whalen, 1996; Hall *et al.*, 2008; Kennedy and Meyer, 1996; Kennedy and Becker, 2006; Peine *et al.*, 1995);
- allergies (Kennedy and Meyer, 1996; Kennedy and Becker, 2006);
- fatigue and sleep/wake patterns (Horner *et al.*, 1997; Kennedy and Meyer, 1996; Kennedy and Becker, 2006; O'Reilly, 1995);
- hormonal changes (Kennedy and Becker, 2006; Taylor *et al.*, 1993b);
- drug effects (Kalachnik *et al.*, 1995; Taylor *et al.*, 1993a);
- caffeine intake (Podboy and Mallery, 1977);
- diet and food deprivation (Talkington and Riley, 1971; Wacker *et al.*, 1996).

It is also likely that some psychiatric disorders and mood states may function as establishing operations, and thereby provide a motivational basis for the expression of challenging behaviour maintained by operant processes (Carr *et al.*, 1996; Emerson *et al.*, 1999b).

Depression, for example, may be associated with an unwillingness to participate in educational or social activities, thus establishing such activities as negative reinforcers (i.e. events whose termination is reinforcing). *If* the person has previously learned that challenging behaviours can terminate such aversive events, we would expect an episode of depression to be associated with an increase in challenging behaviour. It is worth noting, again, that depression does not 'cause' challenging behaviour (i.e. is not a sufficient condition for the expression of challenging behaviour). Rather, the occurrence of challenging behaviour is determined by the combination of: (1) the motivational influence of depression in establishing negative reinforcers; and (2) the pre-existence in the individual's repertoire of challenging behaviours which have previously served an escape function. Again, such a conceptualization suggests two complementary approaches to intervention: (1) change the motivating condition (e.g. treat the person's depression); and (2) change the 'functionality' of the person's challenging behaviour.

For example, Lowry & Sovner describe two case studies in which this type of process appeared to be operating (Lowry and Sovner, 1992). In both cases rapid cycling bipolar mood disorder (assessed through detailed behavioural recording of affect and activity) appeared to be closely associated with variations in self-injury (Case 1) or aggression (Case 2). For both cases, however, anecdotal information was presented to suggest that: (1) specific environmental events (demands from care staff) precipitated episodes of challenging behaviour, but only during particular mood states (depression for Case 1, mania for Case 2); and (2) the persons' challenging behaviour may have functioned within such states to terminate or delay such precipitating stimuli.

In a similar manner the association between specific syndromes and challenging behaviour may be linked to the motivational characteristics associated with that syndrome. That is, syndrome-specific motivational characteristics may influence 'what people want'. Challenging behaviours may (for some people in some contexts) represent a functional and adaptive response to ensure they get what they want. For example:

- diagnostic characteristic of autistic spectrum disorders include a strong preference for sameness, predictability, or preoccupation with limited interests. For such individuals, disruption of the opportunity for sameness may be highly aversive and challenging behaviours may come to serve an important role in escaping from or avoiding such disruptions (Clements and Zarkowska, 2000; Machalicek et al., 2008);
- the onset of dementia among people with Down syndrome has been shown to be associated with increased aggression, fearfulness, sadness and sleep problems (Urv et al., 2008). It is possible that increased rates of (functional) aggression may be indirectly associated with dementia through changes in mood states and motivation;
- the dysregulation of appetite and satiety in people with Prader–Willi syndrome has a clear broad and long-term effect on establishing the reinforcing potential of food, and indirectly therefore on the opportunity for challenging behaviours to emerge if they are functional in accessing food (Whittington and Holland, 2004);

- the high rates of challenging behaviour reported among people with Smith-Magenis syndrome appears to be related to the motivational conditions associated with strong preference for adult attention which is characteristic of the syndrome (Taylor and Oliver, 2008).

Social context, parenting and behavioural processes

We have also seen in the previous chapter that the emergence and trajectory of child behavioural difficulties (in general) are strongly associated with broader aspects of the child's social environment (e.g. family socio-economic position) (Broidy et al., 2003; Jenkins, 2008; Maughan et al., 2004; Tremblay, 2000; Tremblay et al., 2004; Tremblay, 2006), and that parenting practices and behaviours constitute *one* of the key pathways through which this association appears to be mediated (Bradley and Corwyn, 2002; Conger and Conger, 2002; Conger and Donnellan, 2007; Linver et al., 2002). For example, considerable evidence suggests that moderately strong relationships exist between indicators of socio-economic position and such parenting practices and behaviours as: the total amount of speech directed toward children, maternal responsiveness to child initiated speech, access to stimulating material and activities, the use of reasoning with children, harsh, authoritarian and inconsistent parenting, and the physical punishment of children (Bornstein and Bradley, 2003; Fabian Commission on Life Chances and Child Poverty, 2006; Ghate and Hazel, 2002; Seccombe, 2007).

A number of models have been proposed to account for the association between family socio-economic position and parenting practices. These include both Family Stress Models (Conger et al., 1992; Conger and Conger, 2002; Conger and Donnellan, 2007; Emerson and Hatton, in press) and Family Investment Models (Bradley et al., 2001; Bradley and Corwyn, 2002; Davis-Kean, 2005; Linver et al., 2002; Yeung et al., 2002). The Family Stress Model suggests that the effects of poverty on children are mediated through the impact of economic pressures or stresses on parental well-being. Poorer parental well-being is hypothesized to lead both directly to less nurturing and involved parenting and indirectly to the same intermediate outcome via increased parental conflict and reduced warmth/support. Less nurturing and involved parenting is hypothesized to lead to poorer child outcomes. In contrast, Family Investment Models suggest that the link between socio-economic position and child development may be mediated through the increased opportunity of wealthier families to invest in their child's development and future. These models are not, of course, mutually exclusive.

Behavioural models of the emergence and maintenance of challenging behaviour also stress the importance of parenting (at least in the early years) with its focus on the process of 'benevolent enslavement' through the reciprocal social interactions between the people with intellectual disabilities and their primary carers (Guess and Carr, 1991; Kennedy, 2002; Langthorne and McGill, 2008; Oliver, 1993; Oliver *et al.*, 2005; Richman, 2008). What has yet to be investigated, however, is whether parenting behaviours that may increase the risk of the emergence or persistence of challenging behaviour in children with intellectual disabilities are related to socio-economic position.

However, several studies have drawn attention to the association between broad aspects of family functioning and behavioural difficulties in children with intellectual disabilities (Chadwick *et al.*, 2008; Emerson, 2003c; Hardan and Sahl, 1997; Wallander *et al.*, 2006). In addition, there is some limited evidence to suggest that the association between socio-economic position and parenting practices reported in the general population (lower rates of praise, less reciprocation, higher rates of negative behaviours toward the child) is also evident among parents of children with intellectual disabilities (Floyd and Saitzyk, 1992). Given this, it is possible that socio-economic based variations in these parenting practices may, at least in part, account for the observed socio-economic based variations in the emotional and behavioural difficulties of young children with intellectual disabilities.

Broader aspects of the person's social context may also serve to alter children's motivational states in a manner that could help create the conditions for the emergence and persistence of (functional) challenging behaviour. Thus, for example, cumulative exposure to life events or exposure to specific life events such as abuse or parental death may have significant effects on reinforcing properties (positive and/or negative) of social contact. Under conditions in which the person has no more effective means of accessing (or avoiding) social contact, challenging behaviour may emerge.

Possible biological, behavioural and environmental influences on the emergence and persistence of challenging behaviour

Little is known regarding the processes responsible for the early development of challenging behaviour in people with severe intellectual disabilities. We do know, however, that:

- markedly greater rates of emotional and behavioural difficulties are seen in pre-school children with developmental delay when compared with their peers (Baker *et al.*, 2002; Emerson and Einfeld, 2010; Merrell and Holland, 1997; Plomin *et al.*, 2002);
- that the prevalence and persistence of these difficulties are related to family socio-economic position (Emerson and Einfeld, 2010; Emerson *et al.*, in preparation) and specific genetic syndromes (see Chapter 4); and
- that such difficulties are highly persistent across childhood (Einfeld *et al.*, 2006).

The following accounts are, therefore, primarily speculative. However, we believe it likely that to understand the emergence and persistence of challenging behaviour in children with intellectual disabilities it will be important, *in the specific developmental context provided by intellectual disabilities*, to address separately factors associated with the emergence and occurrence during development of repetitive, potentially injurious or minor aggressive/tantrum behaviours and factors associated with their persistence over time (Berkson and Tupa, 2000; Guess and Carr, 1991; Kennedy, 2002; Langthorne and McGill, 2008; MacLean *et al.*, 1994; Murphy *et al.*, 1999a; Oliver, 1993; Oliver *et al.*, 2005; Richman, 2008).

Emergence

In both non-disabled children and in children with intellectual disabilities, repetitive movements commonly occur at transition points in motor development. Thus, for example, rocking on hands and knees occurs prior to the onset of crawling. A number of studies have also indicated that head banging occurs in up to 20% of non-disabled children between the age of 5 and 17 months (de Lissovoy, 1962; Werry *et al.*, 1983), possibly in response to ear infections or teething (de Lissovoy, 1963). As most parents will know, tantrums, aggression and property destruction are common in non-disabled children, reaching a peak at 2 to 3 years of age, after which, for most children, they gradually diminish in both severity and frequency (Broidy *et al.*, 2003; Cairns *et al.*, 1989; Cummings *et al.*, 1989; Loeber and Hay, 1997; Nagin and Tremblay, 1999; Tremblay, 1999; Tremblay *et al.*, 1999; Tremblay, 2000; Tremblay *et al.*, 2004).

The specific developmental context provided by having an intellectual disability may be important in a number of ways.

- Children with severe intellectual disabilities may, as a result of their slower pace of development, exhibit behaviours that are developmentally appropriate, but inappropriate to their chronological age (and may become challenging due to the child's size). They may also exhibit such behaviours for a longer period of time (MacLean *et al.*, 1994).

- Genetic syndromes associated with intellectual disabilities may increase an individual's vulnerability to developing particular behaviours through their influence on the expression of 'uncommitted' (pre-operant) behaviours and on establishing the reinforcing properties of stimuli (Langthorne and McGill, 2008) .

- Similarly, specific disorders that are more common among young children with people with intellectual disabilities (e.g. feeding difficulties, autism) may be associated with difficulties in establishing bonding with carers and an increased risk of experiencing common events (e.g. eating, interactions with carers) as stressful and/or aversive.

- Finally, the socio-economic patterning and social consequences of intellectual disability may put the child at greater risk of experiencing adverse life events (Hulbert-Williams and Hastings, 2008). These may, again, help establish common events as stressful or aversive.

The above points illustrate the potential for very minor or proto 'challenging behaviours', whose expression may well be part of the normal process of development, to occur more commonly, with a greater severity and/or for a longer period of time, among children with intellectual disabilities.

Persistence

Studies of the developmental trajectories of challenging behaviour in non-disabled children, however, indicate that – for most children – such proto 'challenging behaviours' diminish in both severity and frequency in relatively early childhood (Broidy et al., 2003; Cairns et al., 1989; Cummings et al., 1989; Loeber and Hay, 1997; Nagin and Tremblay, 1999; Tremblay, 1999; Tremblay et al., 1999; Tremblay, 2000; Tremblay et al., 2004). For example, the prevalence with which 'typically developing' children in the UK's Millennium Cohort Study score in the 'abnormal' range on the Strengths and Difficulties questionnaire (Goodman, 1999) drops from 31% at age 3 to 9% at age 5, a 71% reduction in prevalence (unpublished data). These marked reductions in rates of conduct difficulties in young children appear to be related to a number of factors including the rapidly developing capacity of the child in areas of problem solving, verbal communication, self-regulation and independence, developments facilitated by the use of effective parenting and behaviour management strategies (Loeber and Hay, 1997; Tremblay, 2000). As we have noted above, however, these gains are inequitably distributed with children living in poorer families and communities being the least likely to benefit.

Again, the specific developmental context provided by having an intellectual disability may be important in a number of ways.

- Most obviously, poorer intellectual ability is likely to be associated with slower development of those capacities, skills and abilities associated with greater problem solving, self-regulation and independence.
- In addition, specific impairments associated with the child's severe intellectual disability (e.g. specific sensory impairments, specific language delay, physical disabilities, problems with impulse control) may result in the child having an additionally restricted behavioural repertoire. Particularly relevant may be the occurrence of restricted receptive and expressive communication skills among children with severe intellectual disabilities (Sigafoos, 2000).
- Increased risk of exposure to lower socio-economic position may further impede development through exposure to less effective parenting strategies (Floyd and Saitzyk, 1992) and reduced opportunities to access developmentally advantageous materials, activities and events.

- Finally, exposure to and experience of overt discrimination (e.g., bullying) and social exclusion that results from systemic or institutionalized discrimination may further reduce the opportunity to access developmentally advantageous materials, activities and events and represent a continuing source of adversity to people with intellectual disability (Emerson, in press).

The likely upshot of these processes is that, as a result of difficulties in developing constructive and efficient alternative to challenging behaviour, children with intellectual disabilities may show both higher initial rates of proto-challenging behaviours and greater persistence of these proto-challenging behaviours over time. There are few data on the latter issue. However, the prevalence with which children with developmental delay in the UK's Millennium Cohort Study score in the 'abnormal' range on the Strengths and Difficulties questionnaire drops from 55% at age 3 to 22% at age 5, a 60% reduction in prevalence (unpublished data).

If children with intellectual disabilities do show both higher initial rates of proto-challenging behaviours and greater persistence of proto-challenging behaviours over time, this provides greater opportunity for alternative maintaining mechanisms to come into play. Thus, for example, the 'comforting' reaction of carers to stress induced tantrums may, over time, come to play an important role in maintaining the behaviour. That is, behaviours which emerge as part of a normal developmental process may, at a later stage, come to be maintained by operant processes time (Guess and Carr, 1991; Kennedy, 2002; Langthorne and McGill, 2008; MacLean et al., 1994; Murphy et al., 1999a; Oliver, 1993; Oliver et al., 2005; Richman and Lindauer, 2005; Richman, 2008). The reciprocal nature of these processes may then, through a process of shaping, act to select more extreme, abnormal and severe variants of the initial behaviour (Carr et al., 1991; Oliver, 1993; Oliver et al., 2005; Taylor and Carr, 1993).

8

The bases of intervention

In this chapter we will address some of the general characteristics of current 'best practice' in approaches to supporting people with intellectual disabilities and challenging behaviour. We will argue that, wherever possible, interventions should be constructional, functionally based, socially valid and, of course, ethical.

The constructional approach

Israel Goldiamond, in one of the classic contributions to the development of applied behaviour analysis, identified two broad orientations which character-ize most approaches to intervention (Goldiamond, 1974). First, he identified a *pathological* approach which focuses on the elimination of behaviours (e.g. self-injury) or states (e.g. anxiety, distress). As he pointed out:

such approaches often consider the problem in terms of a pathology which, regardless of how it was established, or developed, or is maintained, is to be eliminated.

He contrasted this with what he termed a *constructional* approach, an orientation:

whose solution to problems is the construction of repertoires (or their reinstatement or transfer to new situations) rather than the elimination of repertoires (Goldiamond, 1974).

Take, for example, John, a young man with severe intellectual disabilities who displays aggression when attempts are made to teach him new skills. A patho-logical approach would pose the question: how can we stop John being aggres-sive? A constructional approach would formulate the problem in terms of: how can we support John in responding more appropriately to the types of situations which evoke his aggression? As can be seen, while the pathological approach is simply concerned with the *elimination* of aggression, the constructional approach is concerned with the *establishment* of new ways of acting that would be more appropriate in the situations that currently evoke his aggression.

Challenging Behaviour, 3rd edn, ed. Eric Emerson and Stewart L. Einfeld. Published by Cambridge University Press. © E. Emerson and S. L. Einfeld 2011.

There are at least three good reasons for adopting a constructional approach (Cullen *et al.*, 1981). First, as Goldiamond (1974) argued, constructional interventions may be more consistent with notions of human rights. Certainly an approach based on the development of personally and socially appropriate alternative ways of acting would appear to offer some safeguards against the more blatant examples of the abuse of therapeutic power.

Second, most basic and applied behavioural research, the evidence base underlying applied behavioural approaches, has focused on ways of supporting the learning of new skills. This, in effect, provides a very strong empirical foundation for constructionally based interventions.

Finally, a successful pathological intervention *must* involve a constructional component. If a particular behaviour is eliminated, other behaviour(s) are likely to take their place. These replacement behaviours may be positive adaptive responses to the person's situation. Alternatively, they may be other challenging behaviours (the replacement of one challenging behaviour by another is sometimes referred to as 'symptom substitution'). Behaviour is a dynamic process and (like nature) abhors a vacuum. On the face of it, a pathological orientation leaves this aspect of the intervention process to chance. A constructional intervention addresses it directly. Some of the potential benefits of doing so are demonstrated in a study in which Sprague and Horner examined the effects of a pathological intervention and a constructional intervention on the aggression and tantrums shown by Alan, a 15-year-old boy with intellectual disabilities (Sprague and Horner, 1992). Assessment had indicated that his aggression and tantrums were maintained by a process of negative reinforcement, in that they elicited teacher help when he was presented with a difficult task. Each intervention was applied in sequence to only one of Alan's challenging behaviours, his hitting out. While the pathological intervention (verbal reprimands and response blocking) markedly reduced his hitting out, other problem behaviours (head and body shaking, screaming, hitting objects and putting his hands to his face) all increased so that, overall, there was no change in the total rate of challenging behaviours. The constructional intervention (prompting Alan to ask for help in response to difficult tasks) eliminated all problem behaviours, a result which was maintained after 2 months. Given the risk of response covariation or symptom substitution in response to intervention (Schroeder and MacLean, 1987), an approach that centres upon the introduction of alternative behaviours has much to offer.

There will, of course, be situations in which it is easier, simpler, more effective and more ethical to adopt a pathological rather than a constructional approach. Consider, for example, the case in which challenging behaviour only occurs in response to a particular situation which is not itself particularly important for the person's health, development or quality of life (e.g. travelling to school by a particular route (Kennedy and Itkonen, 1993)). An unobtrusive, potentially effective and highly ethical pathological approach to such a situation would be to simply avoid the situation which elicits challenging behaviour. Whether an approach is constructional or not is one of the dimensions that should be considered. It is not, however, the only consideration.

The functional perspective

Perhaps the single most significant development in behavioural practice in relation to intellectual disabilities during the 1980s was the re-emergence of a *functional approach* to analysis and intervention (Carr *et al.*, 1990a; Mace *et al.*, 1991). This approach is based on a belief that *the selection or design of approaches to intervention should reflect knowledge of the causal and maintaining factors underlying the person's challenging behaviour*. Such a belief is, of course, axiomatic to much medical practice. If we are interested in moving beyond symptomatic relief, diagnosis must precede treatment. Indeed, a similar concern with analysis providing the foundation for intervention was evident in the earlier days of applied behaviour analysis. In the intervening period, however, 'behaviour modification' took precedence. As Mace and Roberts point out this approach:

relied largely on [the use of] potent reinforcers or punishers to override the reinforcement contingencies or biologic processes that maintained problem behavior. The treatments were effective, but they were often artificial, conspicuous, difficult to implement for long periods of time, and deemed unacceptable by some caregivers (Mace and Roberts, 1993).

They were also primarily pathological in orientation. The significance of adopting a functional approach can be simply illustrated by considering the use of time-out procedures. The logic of such procedures is that, by arranging the person's environment to ensure that occurrence of challenging behaviour reliably results in reduced opportunity for reinforcement, challenging behaviour should become less frequent over time. Indeed, this is the most likely outcome if time-out were applied to a challenging behaviour maintained by positive reinforcement (e.g. contingent adult attention). In such a case, the time-out procedure would effectively combine extinction (preventing access to adult attention) with a temporary reduction in the background rate of reinforcement. But what would happen if the person's challenging behaviour was maintained by negative reinforcement (e.g. escape from aversive tasks or unwanted attention)? In this case, application of a traditional 'time-out' procedure would guarantee that each episode of the challenging behaviour was (negatively) reinforced by the contingent removal of aversive materials and/or attention (e.g. teacher demands). At best, such an intervention would be ineffective, at worst it could lead to a significant strengthening of the behaviour (Durand *et al.*, 1989; Solnick *et al.*, 1977).

Certain approaches to intervention, including much of the emerging technology of positive behavioural support (see below), are dependent for their success on accurate knowledge about the factors that maintain an individual's challenging behaviour. Those approaches that can be applied in the absence of knowledge of underlying processes tend to be either relatively ineffective (e.g. simple differential reinforcement procedures), or procedurally unacceptable in many contexts (e.g. punishment). Indeed, one of the potential benefits of adopting a functional approach is that it may lead to a reduced reliance on more intrusive methods.

The discussion in the preceding chapter regarding the potential complexity of underlying mechanisms indicates that the adoption of a functional approach may be demanding in that:

- there is no clear link between the topography and function of challenging behaviour. Indeed, very similar topographies shown by the same person may serve different behavioural functions;
- the maintaining factors underlying a person's challenging behaviour may vary over time and across contexts;
- challenging behaviours may be multiply controlled by different contingencies of reinforcement and may reflect a combination of biological and behavioural processes.

The viability of this approach, therefore, lies in the availability of reliable, valid and user-friendly approaches to assessment. This issue will form the basis for the next chapter.

Social validity

In Chapter 2 we introduced the notion of social validity. An intervention which is socially valid should (a) address a socially significant problem; (b) in a manner which is acceptable to the main constituencies involved; and (c) result in socially important outcomes or effects. In that chapter some time was spent discussing the social significance of challenging behaviours and approaches to measuring the 'meaningful outcomes' of intervention. We will return to the latter topic in the next chapter.

The emergence of positive behavioural support

These three trends came together in a very distinct manner with the emergence out of applied behaviour analysis of the discipline of 'positive behaviour support' (Carr et al., 1999; Carr et al., 2002; Carr, 2007; Koegel et al., 1996), a development marked in 1999 by the launch of the new Journal of Positive Behavior Interventions.

Carr (2007) has recently described the primary vision of positive behaviour support in the following terms:

Positive behavior support is ... predicated on the notion that creating a life of quality and purpose, embedded in and made possible by a supportive environment, should be the focus of our efforts as professionals. Our chief concern is not with problem behavior, and certainly not with problem people, but rather with problem contexts. ... Our job is to redesign the counter-productive and unfair environmental contexts that so many people, with and without disabilities, have to contend with in their everyday lives. Our job is to give people the skills, the coping strategies and the desire to deal with the frustration that is an inevitable part of life ...

Much of the content of the following chapters will address the methods and procedures associated with positive behaviour support.

9

Intervention: assessment and formulation

Approaches to assessment that take account of the issues discussed in the previous chapters will need to address a number of factors. First, adopting a functional perspective implies that a key task of assessment will be to identify the processes, behavioural or otherwise, responsible for maintaining the person's challenging behaviours. This process will be referred to as *functional assessment*. Second, taking a constructional approach to intervention suggests that it will be necessary to evaluate aspects of the individual's existing abilities and skills and to identify their preferences and potential reinforcers that may be employed in establishing new behaviours. Finally, the requirement that interventions be ethical and socially valid indicates the need to evaluate the feasibility and potential risks, costs and benefits of the intervention process.

Functional assessment

In recent years a number of reviews and practical guides have focused on the procedures and techniques that may be involved in functional assessment (Carr *et al.*, 1994; Demchak and Bossert, 1996; Durand, 1990; Feldman and Griffiths, 1997; Hanley *et al.*, 2003; Matson and Minshawi, 2007; Matson and Nebel-Schwalm, 2007; O'Neill *et al.*, 1997). In the following sections some of the key issues and trends in this area will be discussed. The process of conducting a comprehensive functional assessment may be conceptualized as comprising four interlinked processes.

1. The selection and definition of challenging behaviours as potential targets for intervention.
2. A *descriptive analysis* of relationships between challenging behaviour, environmental events and biobehavioural states.
3. The generation of hypotheses concerning the nature of the processes maintaining the person's challenging behaviours and the establishing operations and discriminative stimuli which set the occasion for challenging behaviour to occur.

Challenging Behaviour, 3rd edn, ed. Eric Emerson and Stewart L. Einfeld. Published by Cambridge University Press. © E. Emerson and S. L. Einfeld 2011.

4. Possibly, the further evaluation of these hypotheses prior to intervention through *functional analysis.*

It is important to see these aims as interlinked processes, rather than as distinct stages. The relationship between hypothesis formulation and data collection is not linear. Descriptive analyses are themselves based upon hypotheses regarding the kinds of processes that may underlie challenging behaviours. One cannot just 'observe'. The results of descriptive and experimental analyses are likely to feed back into refining the definition of behaviour. Nevertheless, for the sake of simplicity, these four areas will be addressed separately in the sections below.

The identification and definition of behaviours

Four issues need to be considered in relation to the identification and definition of behaviours:

1. the selection of targets for intervention on the basis of their personal and social impact;
2. the importance of assessing the function of separate forms of challenging behaviour;
3. the inclusion within the assessment process of functionally equivalent behaviours; and
4. choice of the unit of assessment.

Selecting socially valid targets for intervention

If interventions are to be socially valid, then the selection of target behaviours should reflect their personal and social significance. That is, they should include those behaviours which, if reduced, would result in the most socially significant (or 'meaningful') outcomes. This will require an assessment of the extent to which the challenging behaviour(s) shown by the person have, or are likely to have, a direct impact upon such factors as:

- the short- and medium-term physical risk to the person and others;
- the restriction of access to functional age-appropriate community-based activities;
- exclusion from their family or community-based services;
- stress and strain experienced by carers and care staff;
- the quality of relationships between the service user and others;
- the need for more restrictive management practices (e.g. restraint, sedation, seclusion).

Unfortunately, this area has received scant attention. While attention has been drawn to the importance of these issues and to some *general* measurement strategies outlined (Evans and Meyer, 1985; Meyer and Janney, 1989; Meyer and Evans, 1993), no structured approaches are currently available that seek to identify the broader impact of the person's challenging behaviour in their particular context.

The form and function of behaviour

The selection and definition of intervention targets should also be guided by knowledge about the potential types of relationship that may exist between behaviour and maintaining processes. As discussed in Chapter 5, the relationship between the form and function of challenging behaviours is far from straightforward. Maintaining factors may be complex, will vary significantly across individuals and may vary within individuals over contexts and time (Lang *et al.*, 2008; Lang *et al.*, 2009a). It is also possible that different forms or topographies of the person's challenging behaviour may be maintained by different processes (Derby *et al.*, 1994; Emerson *et al.*, 1995; Richman *et al.*, 1998; Sigafoos and Tucker, 2000).

This has considerable implications for the selection and definition of target behaviours. It strongly suggests that the assessment process should aim to identify the function of each topographically distinct form of challenging behaviour shown by the individual, rather than aggregate challenging behaviours together under such general terms as 'self-injury' or 'aggression'. The latter option runs the risk that the results of the assessment process may be contaminated by summing together behaviours that are maintained by different processes. This may result in apparently undiscriminated patterns of responding in the results of assessment. Alternatively, it may overlook the functions of behaviours that occur at a relatively lower rate.

One of the tasks of assessment is to identify relationships *between* behaviours (technically, to identify which behaviours belong to which response classes). This can only be achieved, of course, if assessment begins by defining the separate and topographically distinct forms of challenging behaviour shown by the person. Whether to aggregate behaviours together into larger units is an empirical issue that will be determined by the results of the assessment process.

Including functionally equivalent behaviours in the assessment process

A focus on the function, rather than the form, of behaviour also draws attention to the potential value of including behaviours in the assessment process that may be functionally equivalent to the targeted challenging behaviour. This has two possible advantages. First, if it is possible to identify existing socially appropriate functionally equivalent behaviours, these may be used during intervention to substitute for, and displace, the target behaviour (Carr *et al.*, 1994).

Second, it may increase the opportunity for examining aspects of the contextual control of low frequency challenging behaviours. Functional assessment (and, in particular, experimental functional analysis) are often problematic when applied to behaviours that occur at a very low rate. In such instances, it may be possible to identify members of the same response class which occur at a higher rate than the challenging behaviour. This would then allow us to examine the contextual control of the more frequent behaviours as indicators for the main intervention target. For example, a preliminary descriptive analysis may suggest that screaming (which occurs relatively frequently) and aggression (which occurs much more rarely) are members of the same response class. That is, they both appear to be controlled by the same contingencies (e.g. escape from aversive social contact). Assessment could then proceed by gathering more detailed information on the contextual control of the person's screaming as a proxy indicator for aggression. At the end of the day, of course, it would be necessary to demonstrate, rather than simply assume, the applicability of hypotheses generated from descriptive and functional analyses of such proxy indicators to the target behaviour of interest.

Richman and colleagues provide an illustration of such an approach in the functional analysis of aggression shown by three children with intellectual disabilities (Richman *et al.*, 1999). During initial experimental functional analyses, aggression either did not occur or occurred sporadically at extremely low rates. However, less severe challenging behaviours (disruption, screaming) were reliably associated with particular assessment conditions (escape from tasks for two participants, access to toys for the third). Subsequent analysis indicated that aggression was, in fact, a member of the same response class as the less severe forms of challenging behaviour.

The unit of assessment
The functional classification of behaviours also has implications for the size of the behavioural 'unit' selected for analysis. As Scotti and colleagues pointed out, there is probably no greater truism in psychology than 'behaviour consists of a complex stream within which elements are defined and abstracted by the human observer' (Scotti *et al.*, 1991a). Obviously, the way in which we abstract units or chunks of behaviour for the purpose of assessment may have significant implications.

A functional approach will attempt to abstract units on the basis of their functional integrity. That is, it will aim to identify chunks of behaviour that are controlled by their end-point maintaining consequences. So, for example, the sequence of behaviours involved in making a cup of coffee, including all behaviours from getting up to go to the kitchen to sitting down with a freshly brewed cup of coffee, is probably, for most of us, a single functional unit controlled by the reinforcing consequences of coffee drinking. This is only the case, however, if the chain of behaviours is under the control of a specific end-point contingency. In a teaching programme to make coffee, of course, this may not be the case. In such instances this larger sequence may be composed of any number of separate functional units, each controlled by, for example, instructor praise or, alternatively, escape from instructor prompts.

Applying this approach to the identification of challenging behaviours does mean that we need to be constantly aware of the possibility that the composition of functional units containing challenging behaviours may vary across individuals and settings. While for one person a blow to the face may consist of a functional unit maintained by social attention, for another person the functional unit may consist of a complete 'tantrum' of which self-injury is but one part. Hall and Oliver illustrated this point with regards to the self-injurious behaviour shown by a 28-year-old man with severe intellectual disabilities (Hall and Oliver, 1992). They presented descriptive data that indicated that high-rate bursts of self-injury were maintained by positive social reinforcement. No such relationship was apparent, however, when they examined the relationship between low-rate bursts or single occurrences of self-injury and carer attention. There are, of course, plausible reasons to suggest that issues such as behavioural rate, intensity and the presence of concurrent behaviours may be important in defining functional units or operants.

Summary

In summary, then, it has been suggested that:

- the targets for intervention (of which assessment is the first stage) should be primarily guided by the current personal and social impact of the behaviours and the possibility of bringing about more widespread change as a result of successful intervention;
- a key aim of assessment is to identify which of the challenging behaviours shown by the person belong to which response classes. As such, it is important that assessment begins by identifying the behavioural function associated with individual behaviours;
- there may be practical value in including in the assessment process behaviours which may be functionally equivalent to the primary targets of intervention;
- the definition of the target behaviours should aim to capture a functionally integrated unit of behaviour, the nature of which is likely to vary between people and, possibly, across contexts.

Descriptive analyses

The primary objective of a *descriptive analysis* is to identify the processes responsible for maintaining the person's challenging behaviour. It differs from techniques of *experimental functional analysis* (see below) in that it does not involve the systematic manipulation of environmental variables in order to demonstrate experimental control over the person's challenging behaviour. The value of informant-based approaches will be considered first, followed by an examination of the use of more complex observational methods. It will be shown that, while informant-based approaches are simple to administer and provide comprehensive preliminary information, concerns regarding the accuracy of informant reports suggest that they may need to be combined with more detailed observational or even experimental methods in order to arrive at reliable and valid conclusions.

Informant-based approaches
Structured and semi-structured interviews
Structured and semi-structured interviews with key informants are the most widely used approach to the descriptive analysis of challenging behaviour (Desrochers et al., 1997). They are easy to conduct and can provide a wealth of information on a broad range of topics of direct relevance to both the primary and secondary objectives of a functional assessment. Indeed, their use should be considered a logical prerequisite to more complex observational and/or experimental approaches. A number of structured approaches to collecting information from third parties are now available (Carr et al., 1994; Carr et al., 2008; Demchak and Bossert, 1996; Donnellan et al., 1988; Durand and Crimmins, 1988; Durand, 1990; Feldman and Griffiths, 1997; Hanley et al., 2003; Matson et al., 1999; Matson and Minshawi, 2007; Matson and Nebel-Schwalm, 2007; McAtee et al., 2004; O'Neill et al., 1997).

O'Neill and colleagues, for example, describe the use of a structured interview for collecting information from key informants in relation to:
- the topography, frequency, duration, intensity, impact and covariation of the person's challenging behaviours;
- potential setting events (e.g. medications, medical complaints, sleep cycles, eating routines and diet, daily schedule of activities, predictability, control and variety of activities, crowding, staffing patterns), which may be correlated with general variations in the probability of occurrence of the challenging behaviours;
- specific events or situations (e.g. time of day, setting, activity, identity of carer) which are predictive of either high or low rates of occurrence of the challenging behaviours;
- the environmental consequences of the challenging behaviours;
- the efficiency of the challenging behaviours in relation to physical effort, rate and delay of reinforcement;
- alternative communicative strategies used by the person in the context of everyday activities;
- potential reinforcers;
- existing functionally equivalent behaviours;
- the history of previous approaches to intervention (O'Neill et al., 1997).

In addition to these topics, it may be desirable for the clinical interview to cover such issues as:
- the resources (human and material) available in the settings in which challenging behaviours occur;
- staff beliefs about the causes and/or functions of the person's challenging behaviour;

- the pattern (including its consistency) of the physical and emotional responses of staff to episodes of challenging behaviour;
- informal strategies adopted by staff to prevent the occurrence of challenging behaviour.

Structured interview formats are of considerable value in providing a series of prompts to guide the process of behavioural interviewing and, as noted above, they are undemanding of resources and capable of addressing a broad range of issues. Unfortunately, however, the reliability or validity of information collected with such schedules are unknown (Matson and Minshawi, 2007).

Rating scales

There is evidence that assessment of behavioural and emotional difficulties produces the most information when a combination of structured and unstructured approaches to interviewing is used (Cox and Rutter, 1985). Einfeld and Tonge compared descriptions of behaviour disturbance elicited by a structured questionnaire with those elicited by non-directive questioning of 70 parents of children with intellectual disability (Einfeld and Tonge, 2002). On average, 35 items were endorsed on the questionnaire compared with 9 offered by the unstructured approach. Further assessment indicated that many of the extra items elicited by the questionnaire were highly pertinent to formulating an understanding of the behaviour problems.

Structured inventories of behavioural difficulties (completed by carers) have a number of advantages (Einfeld and Tonge, 2002):

- Save time in eliciting a comprehensive account of behaviours of potential importance to formulation
- Ensure behaviours are described in terms assessed for their comprehensibility and reliability
- Facilitate routine data collection of behavioural data given the high prevalence of behavioural disturbances in persons with intellectual disability, allowing the natural history of challenging behaviours to be monitored
- Assess the effects of interventions if the inventory is sensitive to change
- Compare severity of behavioural disturbance of an individual with a suitable comparison group (e.g. others of a similar level of intellectual disability, if norms are available).
- Select those whose challenging behaviour is most severe or exceed a cut-off, when the sensitivity and specificity of the cut-off are known. This is valuable when more intensive assessment is a scarce resource, for example.

Structured questionnaires are also of potential utility in service planning, for example in assessing the number of individuals in a service setting, whose challenging behaviours exceed a determined level. For example, in a special school, such data might be used as an indication of the number of school psychologists required.

Structured behavioural inventories also form the backbone of much research in intellectual disability. Examples include epidemiological studies (Einfeld *et al.*, 2006; Emerson and Einfeld, 2010), behaviour phenotype research in comparing behaviours in one cause of intellectual disability with behaviours of a comparison group (Einfeld *et al.*, 2004), and in intervention research (Aman *et al.*, 2002a).

A considerable number of inventories have been developed that potentially provide a structured component to the assessment of challenging behaviours in people with intellectual disability (Charlot and Mikklesen, 2006; Zimbelman, 2005). These vary in the extent and robustness of their documented psycho-metric properties, and vary in their focus. Some are directed towards particular types of challenging behaviours or psychopathology, for example, behaviours suggestive of depression, or in being more general. Here, we will describe three of the more widely used measures, all covering a broad spectrum of challenging behaviours.

The *Aberrant Behavior Checklist* (ABC) (Aman *et al.*, 1985) is a 58-item measure with five subscales. It has been widely used in research, particularly in studies of medication treatments. It has norms for children and adults with moderate to profound intellectual disability. Its factorial validity has been established in institutional, community and education settings. Inter-rater reliability has varied according to type of rater.

The *Developmental Behavior Checklist* (DBC) (Einfeld and Tonge, 1995b) is a 96-item measure with five subscales. Separate versions are completed by parents/carers of children, Teachers and for carers of Adults. It is available in 21 languages. Norms have been developed for children for Australia, the Netherlands, UK, Germany and Finland, and adults in Australia, and are in preparation in the US. It has robust psychometric properties including sensi-tivity to change.

The *Nisonger Child Behavior Rating Form* (NCBRF) (Aman *et al.*, 1996) has 71 items of problem behaviours but also includes 10 items indicative of social competence. It has Parent and Teacher Versions which have shown good correlation. Behaviour problem subscales are similar to those of the Aberrant Behavior Checklist. It has been used in studies of medication effects.

There also exist a number of rating scales that aim to identify the specific behavioural functions of challenging behaviours.

Motivation assessment scale (MAS): Durand and Crimmins described the development of the MAS (Durand and Crimmins, 1988; Durand, 1990; Durand and Crimmins, 1992). This is a 16-item questionnaire, each item of which is designed to ascertain the extent to which challenging behaviour occurs under conditions associated with behaviours maintained by: sensory consequences; positive social reinforcement; positive tangible reinforcement; or negative social reinforcement. While acceptable levels of inter-informant agreement, test–retest reliability and correspondence with the results of more detailed functional analyses were initially reported, more recent evidence questions the utility of the MAS. First, studies investigating the factorial structure of the MAS have provided conflicting results (Bihm *et al.*, 1991; Duker and Sigafoos, 1998; Singh *et al.*, 1993). Second, numerous studies have questioned the reliability of the data generated by the MAS (Duker and Sigafoos, 1998; Kearney, 1994; Newton and Sturmey, 1991; Sigafoos *et al.*, 1994; Spreat and Connelly, 1996; Thompson and Emerson, 1995; Zarcone *et al.*, 1991). Finally, unacceptably low levels of correspondence between the results of the MAS and the results of more detailed, descriptive and experimental analyses have been reported (Emerson *et al.*, 1995; Toogood and Timlin, 1996).

Questions about behavior function (QABF): The QABF is a 25-item rating scale designed to ascertain the extent to which challenging behaviour occurs under conditions associated with behaviours maintained by: negative social reinforcement (escape); positive social reinforcement (attention); positive tangible reinforcement; non-social reinforcement; and pain. The available evidence suggests that the QABF demonstrates adequate psychometric properties, including a five-factor structure, adequate internal consistency and good inter-rater reliability, and convergent validity with the results of experimental functional analyses (Freeman *et al.*, 2007; Matson and Minshawi, 2007; Singh *et al.*, 2009a). A 15-item short form has recently been developed (Singh *et al.*, 2009a).

Contextual assessment inventory for problem behavior (CAIPB): The CAIPB is a 93-item rating scale designed to describe associations between the occurrence of challenging behaviour and: social/cultural factors (negative interactions and disappointments); task/activity characteristics including daily routines; aspects of the physical environment (comfort, change); and biological factors (medication, illness, physiological states). Initial reports suggest that the CAIPB has acceptable test–retest reliability, convergent and predictive validity, but questionable inter-rater reliability (Carr *et al.*, 2008; McAtee *et al.*, 2004).

Concerns regarding the inter-rater reliability of information derived from informant rating scales suggest that: (1) they should be used with multiple informants; (2) levels of agreement/disagreement should be monitored; (3) areas of disagreement should be actively explored; (4) information should be triangulated with that gained from more detailed observational and, possibly, experimental functional analyses.

Observational methods
The use of observational methods in functional assessments raises a number of issues including: the selection and definition of target behaviours, concurrent behaviours and environmental events; the selection of recording methods and sampling strategies; the reliability and validity of observational methods; observer training; the assessment of inter-observer agreement; subject

NAME: Sophie	OBSERVER: Eric	DATE: 9 January 2000
GENERAL CONTEXT: Home		TIME: 4:30 pm

INTERPERSONAL CONTEXT: Sophie was watching TV. Chris walked in and asked her to tidy her room.

CHALLENGING BEHAVIOUR: Sophie begins to moan, shout and stamp her feet.

SOCIAL IMPACT: Chris looked exasperated and walked out muttering to herself. Sophie went back to watching TV.

NAME: Nick	OBSERVER: Eric	DATE: 10 January 2000
GENERAL CONTEXT: Pub		TIME: 4:30 pm

INTERPERSONAL CONTEXT: Nick, Vicky and Sophie are having a coffee. Vicky and Sophie are deep in conversation with each other.

CHALLENGING BEHAVIOUR: Nick begins to moan, shout and stamp his feet.

SOCIAL IMPACT: Vicky looks concerned, pats Nick on the shoulder and included him in the conversation.

Fig 9.1. Examples of index cards used for recording episodes of challenging behaviour during functional assessment. (Modified from Carr *et al.* 1994.).

reactivity; observer drift; and the use of graphical and statistical methods of data analysis (Barlow *et al.*, 2008; Thompson *et al.*, 2000). To review all these issues is beyond the scope of the present book. Instead, discussion will be restricted to an examination of some of the observational methods that have been used in descriptive analyses of challenging behaviours in applied settings.

ABC charts
The most frequently used observational approach to descriptive analysis in clinical practice involves the recording by care staff of descriptions of a sample of occurrences of antecedent (A) events, the target challenging behaviour (B); and consequent (C) events (Desrochers *et al.*, 1997). Carr, for example, suggest using index cards to record occurrences of challenging behaviour (Carr *et al.*, 1994) (see Fig. 9.1).

The data generated by ABC recording may be summarized to provide, depending upon the sampling strategy employed, three types of information. First, they may provide estimates of the rate or probability of occurrence of episodes of challenging behaviour within specified periods of time (e.g. days) or possibly contexts (e.g. sessions of group instruction). Second, they may highlight aspects of environmental context that appear to be common across episodes of challenging behaviour (e.g. being asked to participate in a non-preferred activity). Finally, they may identify general classes of impact that episodes of challenging behaviour may have on ongoing social or other types of activities (Aman *et al.*, 1985) (e.g. withdrawal of requests, comforting attention from care staff). As such, these descriptions of antecedent and consequent events may generate some tentative hypotheses for further investigation and/or provide further information to triangulate with information collected through interviews and rating scales.

In a more structured approach to ABC analysis, Gardner described the use of conditional probabilities over a one month period to identify antecedent conditions which set the occasion for aggression to occur in a young man with intellectual disabilities (Gardner *et al.*, 1984; Gardner *et al.*, 1986). These events included staff reminders, corrections, repeated prompts, demands, praise and teasing by peers. The conditional probability of aggression following such events ranged from 0.01 (aggression following praise) to 0.32 (aggression following teasing). In addition, they collected information regarding a range of potential establishing operations including weekend visits from his family, difficulty in getting up in the morning, the presence of a particular member of staff and arguments with peers prior to arriving at his day programme. Their results indicated that: (1) 81% of all aggressive outbursts occurred on the 43% of days which included one of these settings events; (2) the mean rate of occurrence of the recorded antecedent conditions was 21.7 per day for days including setting events, compared with 8.3 per day on the remaining days; and (3) the overall conditional probability of antecedent events eliciting aggression was 0.17 for days including setting events, compared with 0.07 on the remaining days.

Scatter plots and related techniques
A key aim of descriptive analysis is to identify patterns of variation in the occurrence of challenging behaviour in order to identify possible establishing operations (Carr *et al.*, 2008; McAtee *et al.*, 2004). Touchette and colleagues described the use of a *scatter plot* to identify temporal and contextual variations in the occurrence of challenging behaviour (Touchette *et al.*, 1985). This relatively simple technique involves the graphical display of partial-interval observational data over successive days to identify those times of day or settings associated with high rates of challenging behaviour. That is, all the observer needs to do is record whether or not an episode of challenging behaviour occurred within the designated time period (e.g. 30 min block) or activity. An example scatter plot is illustrated in Fig. 9.2, The use of scatter plots has become relatively common (Desrochers *et al.*, 1997) and may be of considerable value in identifying clear examples of contextual control. They may, however, be of less value in identifying more complex patterns of temporal or contextual variation (Kahng *et al.*, 1998).

Recording John's aggression to others						
Please put a X in the box if John hits, punches or bites anyone during that time period. Just one X, no matter how often it happens in each 30 minute block						
Week Beginning: 7th June 2010						
	Monday	Tuesday	Wednesday	Thursday	Friday	Saturday	Sunday
07:00–07:30							
07:30–08:00		X				X	
08:00–08:30		X	X		X		
08:30–09:00			X		X		
09:00–09:30							
09:30–10:00							

Fig 9.2. Example scatter plot.

Sequential analysis
Some of the problems associated with ABC charts can be resolved by the use of more complex approaches to recording and analysis, which attempt to identify relationships between challenging behaviour and preceding and consequent environmental events (e.g. social contact with carers). For example, Edelson and colleagues used a 10 second partial interval observational procedure to record the occurrence (or not) of self-injurious behaviours and staff demands, denials or punishment for approximately 5 hours for 20 institutionalized young people with intellectual disabilities (Edelson *et al.*, 1983). They reported sharp increases in the rates of staff contact *prior* to episodes of self-injury for 19 of the 20 participants (suggesting that their self-injury may have served the function of escape from social contact). More recently, the use of hand-held computers to capture data has opened up a range of ever more complex research-based procedures for identifying such associations (Emerson *et al.*, 1995; Emerson *et al.*, 1996b; Emerson *et al.*, 1999a; Martens *et al.*, 2008; McComas *et al.*, 2009; Oliver *et al.*, 2005; Pence *et al.*, 2009; Samaha *et al.*, 2009; Thompson *et al.*, 2000; Toogood and Timlin, 1996). Difficulties associated with the use of such procedures include: resource requirements and technical complexity; use in relatively barren settings in which carer responses to challenging behaviour may be inconsistent; the inherent difficulties of using descriptive analyses to identify relatively 'thin' schedules of reinforcement; failure to identify the appropriate functional unit in descriptive analyses; failure to identify distinct response classes among topographically similar behaviours.

Generating hypotheses

The primary objectives of descriptive analyses are to generate hypotheses regarding the processes maintaining the person's challenging behaviour, including the identification of establishing operations that set the occasion for the behaviour to occur. As indicated in the introduction to this chapter, the relationship between hypothesis formulation and data collection is interactive. Descriptive analyses are themselves based on and provide a way of beginning to test out hypotheses regarding the kinds of processes that may underlie challenging behaviours. Nevertheless, a mid-point stage in any functional assessment requires the specification of more precise hypotheses regarding:

- the process(es) responsible for maintaining the person's challenging behaviour(s);
- the contextual control of these processes;
- the inter-relationships between different forms of challenging behaviour shown by the person.

As we have seen, these relationships may be complex. Maintaining factors may vary across behaviours, time and settings. In addition, challenging behaviours may be multiply controlled. It is appropriate, therefore, to attempt to identify the processes underlying each form of the person's challenging behaviours and to examine the extent to which this underlying process is constant across contexts.

Table 9.1 illustrates the types of context–behaviour–consequence relationships which may be indicative of various underlying processes. At times, the triangulation of information from interviews, rating scales and observational methods may be sufficient to establish the credibility of particular hypotheses. At other times, there may be sufficient uncertainty that further assessment is required. This may involve undertaking more detailed observations or tailoring rating scales to specific circumstances. If such measures are insufficient, it may be worth considering the use of experimental functional analyses.

Experimental functional analysis

Experimental functional analyses involve the demonstration, *through the experimental manipulation of environmental conditions*, of the environmental control of challenging behaviour. Experimental control is demonstrated if important aspects of the challenging behaviour (e.g. its rate, duration, intensity) systematically vary as a result of planned environmental changes. The methods employed in functional analyses form a sub-set of single subject experimental designs (Barlow *et al.*, 2008). Most frequently, functional analyses employ either withdrawal designs (Carr *et al.*, 1976) or alternating treatment (multi-element) designs (Iwata *et al.*, 1982).

Table 9.1. Relationships between antecedent events, challenging behaviours and consequent events that may suggest particular underlying processes

---

Socially mediated positive reinforcement

Does the person's challenging behaviour sometimes result in them receiving more or different forms of contact with others (e.g. while the episode is being managed or while they are being 'calmed down') or having access to new activities?

Is the behaviour more likely when contact or activities are potentially available but not being provided (e.g. situations in which carers are around, but are attending to others)?

Is the behaviour less likely in situations involving high levels of contact or during preferred activities?

Is the behaviour more likely when contact or preferred activities are terminated?

Socially mediated negative reinforcement (escape or avoidance)

Do people respond to the behaviour by terminating interaction or activities?

Is the behaviour more likely in situations in which demands are placed upon the person or they are engaged in interactions or activities they appear to dislike?

Is the behaviour less likely when disliked interactions or non-preferred activities are terminated?

Is the behaviour less likely in situations involving participation in preferred activities?

Is the behaviour more likely in those situations in which they may be asked to participate in interactions or activities they appear to dislike?

Positive automatic reinforcement (sensory stimulation, perceptual reinforcement or opioid release)

Is the behaviour more likely when there is little external stimulation?

Is the behaviour less likely when the person is participating in a preferred activity?

Does the behaviour appear to have no effect upon subsequent events?

Negative automatic reinforcement (de-arousal)

Is the behaviour more likely when there is excessive external stimulation or when the individual is visibly excited or aroused?

Is the behaviour less likely when the individual is calm or in a quiet, peaceful environment?

Does the behaviour appear to have no effect upon subsequent events?

The general model of functional analysis is illustrated in the work of Iwata and colleagues. As described in Chapter 5, Iwata used an alternating treatment design to examine the effect of social context on self-injurious behaviour. They recorded the rates of self-injury under four different conditions. The conditions were selected as representing three *general* cases of the types of contexts under which self-injury maintained by operant processes may occur ('social disapproval', 'academic demand' and 'alone') and one control condition. In the *social disapproval* condition, an adult was present throughout, but did not interact with the child except to express concern or mild disapproval (e.g. 'don't do that') on the occurrence of self-injury. It is assumed that self-injury maintained by positive social reinforcement is more likely to occur under this condition. In the *academic demand* condition, an adult was present throughout and encouraged the child to complete an educational task using a graduated (ask–show–guide) prompting procedure. However, the adult withdrew their attention for 30 seconds contingent on the child's self-injury. This condition was assumed to be discriminative for self-injury maintained by negative social reinforcement. In the *alone* condition, no adults or materials were present. This condition was assumed to be discriminative for behaviours maintained by automatic or perceptual reinforcement. The *control* condition consisted of a stimulating environment in which social attention was delivered contingent upon the non-occurrence of self-injury. Each condition lasted for 15 minutes and was presented on at least four occasions, the order of presentation being randomized. Visual inspection of the consistency of responding across conditions was used as evidence of behavioural function.

Over the past decade, this and similar approaches (English and Anderson, 2006; Northup *et al.*, 1991) have been widely used in applied *research* and some university-based treatment programmes (Asmus *et al.*, 2004; Hanley *et al.*, 2003; Kuhn *et al.*, 2009; Kurtz *et al.*, 2003), but have had relatively little impact on wider clinical practice (Desrochers *et al.*, 1997; Matson and Minshawi, 2007).

The potential value of experimental functional analyses are that: (1) they provide a direct method for identifying functional relationships; (2) they require only brief changes to the person's environment, which is of particular value when sustaining systematic environmental changes may be impractical and/or unethical; (3) they are particularly suitable for examining the effects of environmental conditions, which may be important but which only occur rarely in the person's normal setting; (4) they provide a practical method of testing hypotheses regarding the role of establishing operations in the contextual control of challenging behaviour (Kuhn *et al.*, 2009). The use of these procedures does, however, have a number of limitations. They are demanding of resources and expertise and do, even if briefly, involve creating the conditions under which challenging behaviour will occur more frequently. Clearly, the costs involved in conducting an experimental functional analysis need to be balanced carefully against the likely benefits accruing from such an activity.

Summary

In the sections above, some of the more common descriptive and experimental approaches to the functional assessment of challenging behaviour have been reviewed.

Table 9.2 summarizes some of the key advantages and disadvantages of these approaches. As can be seen, there is a clear (and unsurprising) relationship between the ease of use of different approaches and the detail, reliability and validity of the information generated. While structured interviews are easy to use and

Table 9.2. Descriptive and experimental approaches to functional assessment

	Advantages	Disadvantages
Structured interviews	Ease of use Comprehensive Applicable to low frequency behaviours	Unknown (but probably poor) reliability and validity
Rating scales	Ease of use Focus on specific maintaining factors Applicable to low frequency behaviours	Poor reliability and validity
ABC charts	Ease of use Provide some information about event–behaviour–event sequences Applicable to low frequency behaviours	Unknown (but probably poor) reliability and validity
Scatter plot	Ease of use Provide information about broad aspects of contextual control Can be reliable Applicable to low frequency behaviours	Do not provide detailed information of maintaining contingencies Possibly difficult to interpret
Setting event questionnaires	Ease of use Provide easily interpretable information about broad aspects of contextual control Can be reliable Applicable to low frequency behaviours	Do not provide information about maintaining contingencies
Structured partial-interval record	Can be highly reliable Provide detailed information about immediate event–behaviour–event sequences Precise measurement	More demanding of resources Difficult to apply to low frequency behaviours May have difficulty in distinguishing between positive and negative reinforcement, hence questionable validity
Structured real-time record with sequential analysis	Can be highly reliable Provide extremely detailed information about immediate event–behaviour–event sequences	Highly demanding of resources Difficult to apply to low frequency behaviours

Table 9.2. (cont.)

	Advantages	Disadvantages
Standard experimental analysis	Sound statistical basis for decision making Precise measurement Provide experimental demonstration of contextual control Precise measurement	More demanding of resources Difficult to apply to low frequency behaviours May overlook important variables operating in natural environment
Brief standard experimental analysis	Provide experimental demonstration of contextual control Precise measurement	Difficult to apply to low frequency behaviours Limited internal validity May overlook important variables operating in natural environment
Hypothesis-driven experimental analysis	Link to descriptive analyses Provide experimental demonstration of contextual control Precise measurement	More demanding of resources Difficult to apply to low frequency behaviours

comprehensive, the information generated must be treated with caution. While demanding of resources, the combination of descriptive analyses (e.g. scatter plots, structured observation) with hypothesis-driven experimental functional analyses may provide the best chances of generating clear, reliable and valid information.

Of course, functional assessments are often conducted in situations with limited resources and under conditions in which there may be an obvious need to intervene as quickly as possible. In deciding whether to invest more resources and time in further assessment, it is important to keep in mind the aim of the assessment process, to identify the processes maintaining or underlying the person's challenging behaviour. The role of specific techniques is to generate and test hypotheses about potential processes. Thus, the value of any particular approach is determined by its effect in terms of reducing uncertainty about the processes underlying the person's challenging behaviour. At times, these may become painfully obvious through the use of simple descriptive techniques. In such a situation investing additional resources in order to achieve a minimal reduction in uncertainty could not be justified.

In other situations, however, the use of simple descriptive techniques will reveal complex and confusing patterns of contextual control over the person's challenging behaviour. In such instances, to intervene prior to more detailed analysis would be ethically unjustifiable. As was discussed in the previous chapter, failure to match intervention to analysis may be either ineffective or potentially harmful.

Assessing existing skills, competencies and potential reinforcers

The constructional approach looks for solutions to problems in the 'construction of repertoires (or their reinstatement or transfer to new situations) rather than the elimination of repertoires' (Goldiamond, 1974). As a result, three additional aims of an initial assessment will be:

- to evaluate the broad range of skills and competencies the person possesses and to identify any additional impairments that may limit the establishment of new behaviours;
- to identify discrepancies between the person's current behaviour in key situations and what more desirable alternative responses;
- to identify the person's preferences with regard to potential alternative activities.

General competencies

A large number of questionnaires and checklists have been developed to help assess the general competencies or adaptive behaviours of people with severe intellectual disabilities (Hogg and Langa, 2005; Schalock, 1999, 2004; Thompson *et al.*, 2004). In addition to specific instruments, a number of more comprehensive overviews are available to provide guidance to practitioners regarding the assessment of adaptive behaviours (Browder, 1991, 2001), including texts which focus upon the application of such methods to people with challenging behaviour (Carr *et al.*, 1994).

Over 25 years ago, a number of authors began to suggest that challenging behaviours may be conceptualized as examples of socially inappropriate communication strategies (Carr and Durand, 1985a, 1985b; Carr *et al.*, 1994; Donnellan *et al.*, 1984; Durand, 1986, 1990; Evans and Meyer, 1985). Furthermore, as we shall see below, evidence has begun to accumulate to suggest that some challenging behaviours may be rapidly eliminated by providing the individual with an alternative communicative response that serves the same function as the challenging behaviour (see Chapter 11). As such, the evaluation of the person's communicative competencies and style is of particular significance (Sigafoos, 2000; Sigafoos *et al.*, 2007; Stuart, 2007).

Discrepancy analysis

One of the specific aims of a functionally based constructional approach to remediating challenging behaviour is to identify behavioural deficits specific to conditions known to evoke challenging behaviour. Evans and Meyer (1985) suggested that 'discrepancy analysis' be employed to identify skill deficiencies (and hence targets for intervention) associated with the person's challenging behaviour. A discrepancy analysis involves the comparison of the individual's performance in a problematic situation with that of a more competent peer. On the basis of such a qualitative comparison, specific skill deficiencies may be identified as targets for intervention.

Identifying preferences

The establishment or generalization of alternative responses to challenging behaviours may require the identification of activities or materials that are highly preferred by the person. For example, one possible strategy to reduce challenging behaviours maintained by perceptual reinforcement is to teach the use of, and provide access to, preferred materials or activities (see Chapter 11). Of course, a functional assessment may well identify some extremely powerful reinforcers and contingencies – those maintaining the challenging behaviour itself. Approaches to intervention based on the notion of functional displacement seek to use these contingencies to support alternative behaviours (see Chapter 11).

In other situations, however, the reinforcers maintaining the challenging behaviour may be unclear or not readily accessible by other means (e.g. β-endorphin release). In these cases the identification of alternative highly preferred activities assumes a greater significance. There are two main possible approaches for identifying the preferences of people with severe intellectual disabilities: indirect approaches involving informant interviews; and empirical approaches.

Indirect approaches involve soliciting judgements from key informants regarding the person's preference for particular activities. While indirect approaches have an obvious role to play in selecting potential stimuli or activities, more detailed evaluation may be required to check the validity of informant reports (Hatton, 2004; Lancioni *et al.*, 1996; Reid *et al.*, 1999).

Empirical approaches may be used to identify preferences by examining the actual impact that materials or activities have on behaviour (Hatton, 2004; Lancioni *et al.*, 1996; Reid *et al.*, 1999). A number of strategies have been employed to do this, including measuring: approach responses to individual stimuli presented in an array; approach responses in a forced-choice situation; approach responses to materials presented in an array with or without the replacement of chosen stimuli; time allocation under free-operant baselines; the extent to which stimuli presented contingently would increase the rate of motor behaviours for people with profound multiple handicaps. The available evidence suggests that the measurement of approach responses to materials presented in an array without the replacement of chosen stimuli may constitute the most efficient procedure for selecting preferred activities (DeLeon and Iwata, 1996).

Significance of biological factors for assessment and intervention

When planning interventions, it is generally valid to regard behaviours related to biological factors as relatively less under the individual's control than behaviours attributable to learning (Einfeld, 2005). For example, a child with PWS may have rage attacks in which he hits the teacher or breaks furniture when prevented from buying excess food at the school shop. This reaction is extremely difficult for the PWS child to restrain, as it is driven by hypothalamic dysfunction. Consequently, contingent reinforcement strategies to limit this behaviour are likely to have little success. A behavioural strategy likely to be more successful is to remove the PWS child from areas connected with food. For example, arrangements may be made for the PWS child to spend most of the lunch break in the school library. Families of PWS children learn it is best to close off the kitchen and lock the pantry and refrigerator to prevent gorging. In the case of Williams syndrome, it may be frustrating that the individual is reluctant to participate in an activity that involves confronting some stimulus to which the person is phobic. Again, a reward or punishment strategy is not likely to overcome this intense anxiety. Instead, the individual with Williams syndrome is much more likely to be helped by anti-anxiety medication, for example, sertraline or clomipramine. This does not usually eliminate the phobia but often considerably lessens the anxiety associated with it.

It should be understood, however, that people with genetic disorders causing intellectual disability may also have behaviour disturbance attributable to environmental circumstances or learned experience. For example, an adolescent with Fragile X syndrome may have habitually experienced a harsh and inconsistent discipline style at home, an experience associated with vulnerability to the development of conduct disorder (Patterson and Reid, 1984). In this case, the antisocial behaviour would be best addressed as it would in any other child of similar mental age, irrespective of the presence of Fragile X syndrome.

Two challenges present themselves to the assessing clinician. First, the behaviour phenotypes described above concern only a few of the hundreds of causes of intellectual disability. Clinicians cannot be expected to be aware of the behavioural concomitants of all such causes. However, many of these other causes are unusual, even amongst those with intellectual disability. It is prudent nevertheless to seek advice in the literature as to whether a behaviour phenotype has been reliably established for any individual's cause of intellectual disability. Second, those with challenging behaviour may have behaviour disturbance originating from several sources simultaneously. Even a single behaviour may be multiply determined. For example, in the case of the PWS child with rage attacks, these may be driven by hypothalamic dysfunction but also reinforced by inappropriately harsh and inconsistent responses.

There is no substitute for careful and comprehensive evaluation of behaviour problems, examining the potential contribution from a broad range of sources, including biological factors.

Evaluating the potential risks, costs and benefits of intervention

At a number of points throughout the book, attention has been drawn to the need to address the social validity of intervention. It has been argued that:

- challenging behaviour needs to be understood in its social context, including the impact it may have on broader aspects of the quality of life of the person, their family and friends, co-residents and co-workers, care staff and the public;
- socially valid interventions should involve procedures acceptable to the main stakeholders in the intervention process;
- socially valid interventions should result in socially significant outcomes. These need to be framed in a broader social context than is usually the case and may involve a trade-off between procedural acceptability and the speed and magnitude of outcome.

These observations indicate the need for the assessment process to collect information on a range of potential outcomes in order for the risks, costs and benefits of intervention to be thoroughly evaluated. As has been indicated, however, it is important that the process is individualized and focuses upon the *legitimate outcomes of intervention*. This requires, among other things, seeing that the goals of intervention are separated from more general life-planning processes.

Let us take, for example, the situation of a young woman who shows self-injurious behaviour and lives in a small house with two other women with severe intellectual disabilities. None of the women attends any sort of day programme. Indeed, most of the people served by that particular agency have very restricted lives. In terms of lifestyle, the young woman does not stand out from her peers. In this instance, it would appear that her challenging behaviour is not functionally related to her poor lifestyle. Rather, her social and physical isolation stem from the failing of the service agency. It would seem inappropriate, then, to judge the success of an intervention programme to reduce self-injury on the basis of such general lifestyle variables as earned income, social and physical integration.

Fox and Emerson attempted to identify the outcomes of intervention, which were considered particularly salient by a number of stakeholder groups including people with intellectual disability, parents of people with intellectual disability, clinical psychologists, psychiatrists, nurses, managers and direct support workers (Fox and Emerson, 2001). They used this information to develop a toolkit to help people identify and monitor progress toward such 'meaningful outcomes' for people with intellectual disabilities and challenging behaviour (Fox and Emerson, 2002, in press). Lucyshyn and colleagues provide an example of the use of a broad range of measurement approaches to evaluate the social validity of community-based supports for a young woman with life-threatening self-injury (Lucyshyn *et al.*, 1995). They employed a variety of quantitative and qualitative approaches to measure outcomes in such areas as: frequency of self-injury and aggression; participation in community-based activities; activity preferences; social integration; relationships with her family; expressed satisfaction; medication use; and staff turnover.

Summary

In the sections above, some of the key techniques and issues involved in the assessment of challenging behaviour have been examined. It has been argued that the assessment process will need to:
- identify and prioritize socially significant targets for intervention;
- determine the processes underlying the challenging behaviour(s) shown by the person;
- assess general and specific aspects of the person's existing skills and competencies;
- identify preferences;
- collect information that will allow the attainment of the legitimate targets of intervention to be evaluated.

10

Pharmacotherapy

There have been a number of surveys assessing the extent of prescription of psychotropic medication to people with intellectual disability, and whether it has been in keeping with good clinical practice. These surveys have frequently documented high levels of medication use and poor prescribing practice (Matson and Neal, 2009; Rinck, 1998; Spreat *et al.*, 2004). For example, Holden and Gitelson found that 37% of people with intellectual disabilities in one Norwegian county were using psychotropics, that prescriptions frequently violated current guidelines, especially when provided by general practitioners (Holden and Gitlesen, 2004). For example, many prescriptions had not been indicated by a diagnosis, alternatives to medications had rarely been explored and evaluation of effects and side effects were exceptions.

Doctors are often subject to considerable pressure to prescribe medication to diminish or contain challenging behaviours. This is not surprising since psychotropic medications are available that are potent in producing tranquilization, fast-acting, require little expertise on the part of untrained carers, and may be relatively inexpensive compared with behavioural analysis and intervention. Unfortunately, however, psychotropic medications are nearly always associated with unwanted effects, at least in some individuals. These can vary from minor nuisance to life-threatening. The presence of unwanted effects has sometimes led to inappropriately restrictive attitudes towards medication use. In some locales, authorities have been set up to authorize or monitor prescribing of medications, especially psychotropic drugs, to persons with intellectual disabilities. These authorities have varied in their sophistication, understanding and co-operation with or hostility towards, medical practitioners. Thus the prescriber is often caught in the bind of pressure from some quarters to prescribe to relieve a desperate situation and objections to such practice from others.

Consequently, it is important for prescribers to consider the use of drugs in people with intellectual disability in a systematic way. Such approaches, which have been described by a number of authors (de Leon *et al.*, 2009; Deb *et al.*, 2006; Einfeld, 1990; Kalachnik *et al.*, 1998; Szymanski and King, 1999; Unwin and Deb, 2008), are summarized below.

Challenging Behaviour, 3rd edn, ed. Eric Emerson and Stewart L. Einfeld. Published by Cambridge University Press. © E. Emerson and S. L. Einfeld 2011.

General guidelines

1. The decision to prescribe psychotropic medication should follow a comprehensive assessment of the individual's emotional and behavioural health. Such a comprehensive assessment will include not only descriptions of the behaviour, the formulation of precipitating and palliating factors but also an assessment of the efficacy of all the past modes of treatment. The prescriber should try to resist 'knee-jerk' responses, despite the pressure of crisis presentations.

2. Proper consideration should be given to the issue of informed consent, particularly with respect to legal requirements. Frequently, the practitioner is required to make an all-or-none decision with respect to the person's capacity to consent. In fact, capacity will be quite variable. For example, a person with mild intellectual disability may be able to understand that a antipsychotic may make them feel calmer, but not weigh up the advantages of that against the risk of side effects.

3. The psychotropic treatment needs to be an integrated part of other concurrent treatments. It is unusual for psychotropic medication alone to be sufficient treatment. This requires good interdisciplinary communication.

4. The precise target symptoms for which the psychotropic medication is being prescribed should be stated. In other words, what exactly is it hoped the psychotropic medication will treat? It is very difficult to gain reliable information on global impressions, such as 'person will be less disruptive' or 'more compliant'. Better to use specific descriptions such as 'frequency of person hitting others will be less'.

5. One needs to establish some method for reliably and validly documenting changes in the target symptoms during the course of treatment.

6. This record should demonstrate that target symptoms have had a positive response to the medication before the psychotropic medication is continued. While this is obvious, it is common for people to be seen who have been receiving large doses of antipsychotics for many years without any evidence that it's helped their continuing behaviour difficulties.

7. When target symptoms have been reduced or absent for a reasonable period then an attempt should be made to reduce the dose being prescribed. Again reliable and valid measures of the effect of this dosage change should be available. Similarly, people are frequently maintained on medication for lengthy periods, long after symptoms have resolved, out of fear that the behaviours will recur, even though their circumstances have changed.

8. When a psychotropic medication is withdrawn, a proper withdrawal regime should be designed. Withdrawal symptoms appear commonly in this population if long-standing treatments are terminated suddenly. A possible

regime for reducing antipsychotics could be a reduction in daily dose of 20% per month.

9. Because of the presence of organic brain dysfunction, the response to psychotropic drugs is often idiosyncratic. This suggests that small doses should be used initially with close attention paid to the emergence of side effects.

10. In addition to the above, general principles of pharmacotherapy need to be observed as with any other patient, that is, proper attention should be paid to issues of compliance, pharmacokinetics, drug interactions and side effects.

The effectiveness of, and factors in prescribing, particular medications

Antipsychotics

The antipsychotics are the most researched medications in this area, but few studies have been rigorous enough to allow conclusions as to their value for the treatment of psychosis or disruptive behaviour. Deb *et al.* reviewed studies of the effectiveness of antipsychotics in adults with intellectual disability, and found only one randomized controlled trial (Deb *et al.*, 2007). Overall, many studies were uncontrolled case reports, using unvalidated measures, using antipsychotic medications for variable indications including a range of psychiatric disorders and challenging behaviours. Tyrer *et al.* compared rispiridone, haloperidol and placebo administered to adults with intellectual disability and aggressive behaviour (Tyrer *et al.*, 2008). No other assessment of psychiatric or behavioural factors was undertaken. All subjects improved equally. The same group also demonstrated that there was no cost-effectiveness advantage to the antipsychotic treatment when used in this way (Romeo *et al.*, 2009).

In children and adolescents with intellectual disability, however, a number of double-blind placebo controlled trials of risperidone have shown positive results. Aman and colleagues and Snyder and colleagues have reported in children and adolescents with intellectual disability, using doses of 0.02 to 0.06 mg/kg/day (Aman *et al.*, 2002b; Snyder *et al.*, 2002). These studies demonstrated an approximately 50% reduction in challenging behaviours, significantly greater than placebo. Somnolence was transient and there was no impairment of cognition. However, weight gain was common, and prolactin levels were persistently elevated. Whilst these agents cause lower levels of short-term extrapyramidal side effects, there is only limited evidence that the risk of tardive dyskinesia is lessened (Beasley *et al.*, 1999). They are also associated with raised liver enzymes (Benazzi, 1998) but the clinical significance of this is unclear. There is no substantive evidence that the newer antipsychotics have greater efficacy than the traditional ones.

Buzan and colleagues (Buzan *et al.*, 1998) have reviewed 84 published cases of clozapine use in adults with intellectual disability. They concluded that clozapine was both efficacious and well tolerated. It is possible that the haematological side effects of clozapine have led practitioners to be too cautious in utilizing this medication.

Antipsychotic medications frequently cause sedation and compromise cognitive functions and self-help skills (Unwin and Deb, 2008). In addition, extrapyramidal side effects are common. For example, Campbell *et al.* found that 34% of autistic children who were receiving haloperidol over a prolonged period had developed dyskinesias, mostly associated with withdrawal (Campbell *et al.*, 1997; Matson *et al.*, 2010).

Akathisia is an important side effect of antipsychotics to consider in persons with intellectual disability. Persons with limited verbal skills frequently are unable to describe the sense of restlessness and irritability, which can be very distressing. This can lead to increased agitation, which may mistakenly be seen as an indication for increased doses of antipsychotics, making the problem worse. Carers are sometimes very surprised to see a decline in agitation or aggression when antipsychotic dose is reduced. Another rare but important complication of antipsychotic medication is Neuroleptic Malignant syndrome. Boyd (1993) (quoted in Reiss & Aman, 1998)) found the fatality rate (21%) to be double that occurring in persons without intellectual disabilities. Guidelines for the prescription of antipsychotics has been provided by de Leon and colleagues (de Leon *et al.*, 2009).

Antidepressants and electroconvulsive therapy

Depression can be difficult to diagnose with confidence, given the patient's likely limited verbal skills. However, given the safety of selective serotonin reuptake inhibitors (SSRIs), a low threshold for instigation of an antidepressant trial is reasonable. SSRIs have largely supplanted the tricyclic antidepressants in the treatment of depression in this population, given the lesser impact of side effects. Agitation and nausea are the most common. There is inconclusive evidence that one SSRI has any greater efficacy than another. As stated above, it is important to start with small doses and, for this reason, SSRIs which are available in liquid form present advantages in that titration of small doses is easier.

SSRI's have also been widely used in the field to treat perseverative and repetitive behaviours, including rituals of autism, preoccupations in Asperger disorder and self-injurious behaviour. This application was reviewed by Sohanpal *et al.*, who identified only one randomized controlled trial (Sohanpal *et al.*, 2007). Lewis *et al.* found clomipramine to reduce the severity of stereotypy, hyperactivity and irritability. A range of case reports and uncontrolled studies were summarized as indicating that improvements in these symptoms were no more likely than no improvement (Lewis *et al.*, 1995).

Anxiolytics

There have been no specific studies of the treatment of anxiety in persons with intellectual disability. Clinicians have reported improvements in phobic or generalized anxiety disorders as well as obsessive compulsive disorder with treatment with SSRIs similar to that seen in the general population. Moclobemide is an alternative, but in the author's experience has less efficacy than the SSRI's. Buspirone has been described in case reports as of assistance. There is little or no indication for the use of benzodiazapines for the treatment of behavioural and emotional disturbance, although they are commonly used in the treatment of epilepsy. Benzodiazapines, particularly clonazepam, frequently cause disinhibition and irritability in persons with organic brain impairments.

Mood stabilizers

Typical manic depressive illnesses is occasionally seen, but more frequently people with intellectual disability present with instability of mood, that is to say rapid fluctuations between excitement, irritability and high levels of activity alternating with withdrawal and loss of interest. Deb *et al.* have recently reviewed the use of mood stabilizers with persons with intellectual disability, but found only one randomized controlled trial (Deb *et al.*, 2008). Langee (1990) found 42% of individuals treated with lithium improved significantly. Lithium has also been widely used particularly for impulsive aggressive behaviour, though evidence for a particular efficacy for this presentation is equivocal.

It should be noted that hypothyroidism is more common in Down syndrome and that tremors and other movement disorders are more common in individuals with intellectual disability, so particular care is needed to monitor for the side effects of lithium. Arbamazepine and valproate have been widely used as mood stabilizers in children and adolescents with intellectual disability and have lower toxicity risks than lithium. Despite their wide use, there are surprisingly few studies of their use, predominantly case reports. Carbamazepine has the disadvantage of requiring more frequent monitoring of serum level, and SSRIs tend to raise the serum level. Valproate can cause liver disease, especially in younger children, and liver function should be monitored in the initial stages of its use.

Stimulants

The principal indication is for the same purpose as in children without intellectual disability, that is for the treatment of Attention Deficit Hyperactivity disorder. The DSM-IV diagnosis of Attention Deficit disorder requires that the symptoms of inattention or hyperactivity and impulsivity are maladaptive and excessive for the developmental level. There is some evidence to suggest that those with moderate and severe intellectual disability do not respond as well to stimulants as those with mild intellectual disability (Aman *et al.*, 1991). ICD-10 includes Overactive disorder associated with mental retardation and stereotyped movements, a category of uncertain validity. Stimulants may worsen epilepsy, anxiety and tics, all of which are more common in children with intellectual disability.

The SSRIs have fewer side effects than stimulants for the treatment of ADHD, though appear to be somewhat less potent. Clonidine has a calming effect in hyperactivity, though this is often at the cost of sedation, tolerance development and requirements to monitor blood pressure. Curiously, there have been no systematic studies, of which this author is aware, of studying stimulants in Prader–Willi Syndrome, despite their appetite suppressant properties.

Anticonvulsants

Anticonvulsants are frequently prescribed for persons with intellectual disability, either for management of epilepsy or as mood stabilizers as above. Vigabatrin is less used than previously, because it causes visual field defects, and occasional psychosis. It can have marked changes on alertness either by increasing alertness even with improved cognitive function in persons with intellectual disability and severe epilepsy, but can also decrease alertness and awareness. Lamotrigine can also improve alertness, but may also cause decline in cognitive function. It has also been occasionally noted to cause insomnia, irritability or aggression. Topiramate can improve or diminish alertness and cognitive function and this is sometimes quite marked. In addition, it frequently causes nausea and anorexia. Benzodiazepines are also used for epilepsy, but may cause disinhibition or irritability. When a person with intellectual disability and epilepsy presents with these symptoms, it is always worth considering an alternative anticonvulsant if possible.

Antilibidinal agents

Inappropriate sexual behaviours of some adolescents with intellectual disability can cause considerable concern to others and restriction for the individual. Consequently, there has been a growth in use of testosterone antagonists to reduce libido. Cyproterone is now widely favoured as it is active orally, but causes weight gain. LHRH analogues are the most effective and safest method for reducing testosterone levels over prolonged periods, but are expensive and of limited availability. The pharmacological reduction of libido is potentially of some ethical concern. Prescription to this end should only follow efforts to redirect inappropriate sexual behaviour through behavioural and educative means. It may then be that the best interest of the adolescent with intellectual disability is served by suppression of a natural aspect of human function. These issues are discussed in greater detail by Clarke (1989).

Opioid antagoniosts

Opioid antagonists have been used in the treatment of self-injurious behaviour (SIB) in persons with intellectual disability, based on the possibility that such SIB is maintained by disturbance of the beta-endorphin system, so that SIB is pleasurable rather than aversive. There is some evidence to support this notion, especially in association with disruption of the balance between beta-endorphin and adrenocortico-stimulating hormone secretion (Sandman *et al.*, 2008). Naltrexone is the opioid antagonist most used, since it is absorbed orally. Symons *et al.* have summarized results from 27 studies of naltrexone used for the treatment of self-injurious behaviour (Symons *et al.*, 2004). These studies involved 86 participants. Eighty per cent of subjects were reported to have lower levels of SIB relative to baseline during naltrexone administration and, in about half of the subjects, SIB was reduced by 50% or greater. Doses above 1 mg/kg were more effective. For unknown reasons, males were more likely than females to respond. However, some of the studies were case reports rather than controlled studies, and it is unclear whether there was a tendency to under-report negative outcomes.

Summary

The literature on the use of psychotropic medications remains sparse in comparison with that available for the general population. The principal reason for this is that most research in psychopharmacology is funded by pharmaceutical companies. These companies have not regarded the considerable expense of conducting studies with people with intellectual disability as a worthwhile commercial investment, given the limited potential market offered by this population. The one exception of which the authors are aware is the commercial funding of trials of rispiridone in children with developmental disabilities. As a consequence, the literature on the use of risperidone is much more extensive than it is for other later-generation antipsychotics.

The limited literature has a number of consequences. First, there are few studies with randomized controlled trials. As a consequence, the level of evidence for treatment effects is limited. Second, many studies have examined medication use in largely unselected populations of persons with intellectual disability. Given the heterogeneity of people with intellectual disability across biological, psychological and social domains, it would not be expected that psychotropic medications would act in a consistent manner. What the field now requires are studies of individual or comparison medications for either specific symptoms (challenging behaviours) or disorders (e.g. depression), in groups of participants specified in meaningful ways. Examples of meaningful groupings of study participants could be those with challenging behaviours as a consequence of a common aetiology of intellectual disability (behaviour phenotypes), or who have common histories (e.g. non-responders to particular behavioural interventions), or common psychosocial characteristics (e.g. those with mild intellectual disability from socially deprived families). The last example would be in recognition of the need for drug treatments to show effectiveness as well as efficacy.

Third, practitioners will often have to adopt an 'rational/empirical' approach to use of medications. That is, instigate trials of medication after weighing up the likelihood of effectiveness, based on the degree to which the presentation resembles that seen in populations where efficacy has been demonstrated. This estimation then needs to be weighed against the risks of treatment. The effects need to be assessed validly and revisions made accordingly to medication plans.

11

Behavioural approaches

In this chapter a range of behavioural approaches to reducing challenging behaviour will be examined. It is not the intention, however, to provide a comprehensive meta-analysis of this vast area (Ball *et al.*, 2004; Campbell, 2003; Didden *et al.*, 1997; Didden *et al.*, 2006; Harvey *et al.*, 2009; Lang *et al.*, 2009b; Marquis *et al.*, 2000; Scotti *et al.*, 1991b). Instead, attention will be directed to those approaches that form important components of the emerging technology of positive behavioural support (Carr *et al.*, 1999; Carr *et al.*, 2002; Carr, 2007; Koegel *et al.*, 1996).

The contents of the chapter have been organized in terms of the general rationale behind particular approaches to intervention. Thus, approaches will be discussed that are based on: manipulating antecedent stimuli or changing the context to prevent the occurrence of challenging behaviour; behavioural competition or response covariation; disruption of maintaining contingencies; and punishment or other 'default' technologies. In practice, of course, intervention programmes are likely to consist of a number of distinct approaches. The chapter will, therefore, be concluded by an examination of multi-component strategies.

Preventing the occurrence of challenging behaviours through the modification of establishing operations

The results of a comprehensive functional assessment should indicate: (1) contexts or settings in which challenging behaviour is significantly more likely to occur; (2) establishing operations that may either activate or abolish the contingencies maintaining the person's challenging behaviour; and (3) the nature of the contingencies themselves. This knowledge opens up possibilities for either preventing or reducing the occurrence of challenging behaviours by the 'indirect' manipulation of antecedent variables.

As we noted previously, it is rare that challenging behaviours consistently occur in response to particular situations. More commonly, while the behaviour

Challenging Behaviour, 3rd edn, ed. Eric Emerson and Stewart L. Einfeld. Published by Cambridge University Press. © E. Emerson and S. L. Einfeld 2011.

of interest may be more likely to occur in certain situations (e.g. during a specific type of instructional task), its actual occurrence can show considerable variability over time. People have good days and bad days. The identification of establishing operations which account for such variability allows, through their modification, for the development of highly effective non-intrusive approaches to intervention which, in effect, undercut the motivational basis underlying challenging behaviours (Carr, 1988; Carr and Smith, 1995; Carr et al., 1996; Friman and Hawkins, 2006; Kennedy and Meyer, 1998; Kern et al., 2006; McGill, 1999; Smith and Iwata, 1997).

For example, a functional assessment may indicate that a person's aggression is maintained by escape from social demands (Miltenberger, 2006). Further analysis may help identify those establishing operations *which establish demands as aversive stimuli* and, consequently, as negative reinforcers. These could include such diverse factors as fatigue, illness, sedation, hangover, caffeine ingestion, the nature of preceding activities, the presence of preferred competing activities, the pacing or style of demands. The modification of any establishing operations that might be identified could, therefore, prevent social demands acquiring aversive properties and hence reduce aggression by undercutting its motivational base (if demands are no longer aversive why would someone wish to escape from them?). In the study described in Chapter 4 (Carr et al., 1976), rates of self-injury were immediately and significantly reduced by embedding demands in the context of a story. In all probability, these startling results reflect the operation of establishing operations.

As indicated above, a host of variables may influence the extent to which these underlying processes are operational in particular contexts. These include aspects of the individual's bio-behavioural state, preceding interactions and aspects of the current context for behaviour (Luiselli, 2006).

Bio-behavioural state includes such factors as alertness, fatigue and sleep/ wake patterns (Brylewski and Wiggs, 1999; Espie, 1992; Green et al., 1994; Guess et al., 1990; Horner et al., 1997; Kennedy and Meyer, 1996; O'Reilly, 1995), hormonal changes (Taylor et al., 1993b), drug effects (Kalachnik et al., 1995; Taylor et al., 1993a), caffeine intake (Podboy and Mallery, 1977), seizure activity (Gedye, 1989a, 1989b), psychiatric disorders (Emerson et al., 1999b; Lowry and Sovner, 1992), food deprivation (Talkington and Riley, 1971; Wacker et al., 1996), mood (Carr et al., 1996), illness or pain (Bosch et al., 1997; Carr and Smith, 1995; Carr et al., 1996; Gardner and Whalen, 1996; Kennedy and Meyer, 1996; Kennedy and Becker, 2006; Peine et al., 1995; Symons et al., 2008; Symons et al., 2009).

Preceding interactions include such factors as preceding compliance (Harchik and Putzier, 1990; Horner et al., 1991; Mace et al., 1988), task repetition (Winterling et al., 1987), the delay or cancelling of previous activities (Horner et al., 1997), critical comments from others (Gardner et al., 1986), immediately preceding interactions (O'Reilly, 1996; O'Reilly et al., 1999), temporally distant social interactions (Gardner *et al.*, 1986; O'Reilly, 1996), physical exercise (Lancioni and O'Reilly, 1998), the route taken to a setting (Kennedy and Itkonen, 1993), and time of awakening (Gardner *et al.*, 1984; Kennedy and Itkonen, 1993).

The *current context* for behaviour includes such factors as noise, temperature, levels of demand and positive comments from staff (Kennedy, 1994a), location (Adelinis *et al.*, 1997), music (Durand and Mapstone, 1998), crowding (McAfee, 1987), preference and choice regarding concurrent activities (Cooper *et al.*, 1992; Dunlap *et al.*, 1994; Dunlap *et al.*, 1995; Dyer *et al.*, 1990; Ferro *et al.*, 1996; Foster-Johnson *et al.*, 1994; Lindauer *et al.*, 1999; Ringdahl *et al.*, 1997; Vaughn and Horner, 1995; Vaughn and Horner, 1997), the amount of non-contingent reinforcement available in the setting (Derby *et al.*, 1998; Hagopian *et al.*, 1994; Hanley *et al.*, 1997; Roscoe *et al.*, 1998; Vollmer *et al.*, 1993; Vollmer *et al.*, 1995), concurrent social interactions and the nature of surrounding activities (Carr *et al.*, 1976), and the presence of such idiosyncratic variables such as small balls, puzzles and magazines (Carr *et al.*, 1997).

A wide range of antecedent manipulations have been shown to decrease the rate of various types of challenging behaviour. It is probable that many of these have their effect by reducing the potency of the reinforcers responsible for maintaining challenging behaviour. That is, they involve the modification of establishing operations or stimuli that set the occasion for the behaviour to occur. A number of specific techniques and general approaches are outlined below.

Modification of bio-behavioural state

As noted above, a range of bio-behavioural states have been shown to be correlated with the occurrence of challenging behaviour. These include such factors as alertness, fatigue, sleep/wake patterns, hormonal changes, drug effects, seizure activity, psychiatric disorders, mood and illness or pain. Carr *et al.*, for example, report preliminary data to suggest that the pain associated with menses established the negatively reinforcing capacity of staff demands (i.e. make staff demands 'aversive' and thus evoke escape motivated aggression) (Carr and Smith, 1995; Carr *et al.*, 1996). The results of these and other studies suggest that, in some instances, effective reductions in challenging behaviours may be achieved by modification of bio-behavioural states *when such states have been linked through functional assessment to increased rates of challenging behaviour.* Such 'indirect' approaches to intervention could include the treatment of sleep disorders (Durand *et al.*, 1996; Kennedy and Meyer, 1996; Lancioni *et al.*, 1999; O'Reilly, 1995; Piazza *et al.*, 1998), appropriate treatment of medical conditions (Bosch *et al.*, 1997; Kennedy and Meyer, 1996; Peine *et al.*, 1995) and changes to medication regimes (Kalachnik *et al.*, 1995).

Changing the nature of preceding activities

The nature of preceding activities may have a significant impact on people's responses to ongoing events. Krantz and Risley, for example, identified some effects of the scheduling of activities upon disruptive behaviour in a pre-school setting (Krantz and Risley, 1977). They reported that levels of disruption during a story-telling period were markedly reduced if the activity was preceded by a rest period rather than by a period of vigorous activity. In a similar vein, Wahler presented data to suggest that aversive interactions between low-income parents and their relatives or workers from service agencies set the occasion for subsequent aversive interactions between parents and children (Wahler, 1980).

Studies have examined the relationship between a variety of types of preceding activities and subsequent rates of challenging behaviour. These include studies of the effects of: behavioural momentum in increasing compliance and reducing challenging behaviours associated with non-compliance; choice making; task variety and stimulus fading; exercise; and a variety of idiosyncratic establishing operations.

Mace *et al.* described the application of the phenomenon of *behavioural momentum* to the reduction of challenging behaviour (Mace *et al.*, 1988). Behavioural momentum refers to the temporary but marked increase in response probability for a general response class following a period of reinforcement. That is, following repeated reinforcement, behaviour appears to gain a 'momentum', which makes it temporarily resistant to change. They applied the notion of behavioural momentum to increase the compliance of four men with intellectual disabilities. They first identified requests which either elicited high (high probability requests) or low (low probability requests) rates of compliance. They reported that compliance with low probability requests was significantly increased by preceding them with a series of high probability requests. Subsequent studies have also demonstrated that this procedure is effective in reducing challenging behaviours associated with non-compliance. For example, preceding a request to take medication (which often led to challenging behaviour) with a series of requests to 'give me five' resulted in increased compliance and reduced challenging behaviour (Harchik and Putzier, 1990). It would appear that the generalized response class of complying with requests had gained a momentum from prior reinforcement which 'carried over' to the more problematic request. A number of studies since then have illustrated the viability of this procedure across a range of settings (Davis *et al.*, 1992; Horner *et al.*, 1991; Mace and Belfiore, 1990).

Winterling *et al.* reported that increasing task variety (and decreasing repetition) was associated with immediate and significant reductions in aggression and tantrums for three young people with intellectual disabilities and autism (Winterling *et al.*, 1987). These results are consistent with the suggestion that *repeated exposure* to the task within a short period of time acted as an establishing operation, leading to subsequent presentations acting as negative reinforcers. However, Lancioni reported that, while three of four participants with severe intellectual disabilities expressed strong preferences for task variety (over task repetition), the other participant expressed strong preferences for task repetition (Lancioni *et al.*, 1998). As with the results of studies on environmental enrichment, these data highlight the need for interventions to be based on individualized functional assessments.

A small number of studies have examined the potentially therapeutic effects of *stimulus fading* (Heidorn and Jensen, 1984; Kennedy, 1994a). Stimulus fading refers to the temporary withdrawal and gradual re-introduction of stimuli that set the occasion for challenging behaviour. This technique has been combined with the use of negative extinction in the treatment of escape-motivated self-injurious behaviour. The results of these studies suggest that, while stimulus fading may help avoid the occurrence of an extinction burst (Zarcone *et al.*, 1993), it may not necessarily increase the effectiveness of the extinction procedure itself (Zarcone *et al.*, 1993).

The technique of stimulus fading is procedurally similar to the techniques of systematic desensitization and reinforced graded practice in the treatment of fears and phobias. This, suggests that the effectiveness of stimulus fading may be increased if combined with procedures incompatible with arousal (e.g. relaxation, massage, eating). While there have been no tests of this specific hypothesis, a few case studies have reported the beneficial effects of including relaxation training or massage as a component of more complex treatment packages (Bull and Vecchio, 1978; Dossetor *et al.*, 1991). Steen and Zuriff, for example, describe the use of relaxation training and reinforced practice during the phased removal of restraints from a 21-year-old woman with severe intellectual disabilities (Steen and Zuriff, 1977). Prior to intervention, she had been kept in full restraint (involving tying her ankles and wrists to her bed) for the previous 3 years in an attempt to control her self-injurious finger biting, and the scratching of her legs, face and scalp. Within 115 sessions over a total time of 17 hours, her self-injury was virtually eliminated.

Numerous studies have reported that physical exercise may result in reductions in stereotypic, self-injurious and aggressive or disruptive behaviours during immediately subsequent activities. Greater reductions in challenging behaviour have been reported for more strenuous activities (e.g. jogging compared with ball games) (Kern *et al.*, 1984). These results cannot be accounted for by overall reductions in activity, since some studies also report increases in the amount of time spent on task and work performance (Kern *et al.*, 1982). These results may reflect the impact of exercise on dopamine turnover (Schroeder and Tessel, 1994). Whatever the mechanism, the accumulated evidence points to a consistent, although not inevitable, short-term effect of aerobic exercise on subsequent activity (Lancioni and O'Reilly, 1998).

Finally, Horner *et al.* describe the use of *neutralizing routines* to eliminate the effects of establishing operations (Horner *et al.*, 1997). They demonstrated that, for each of three children with severe intellectual disability, their aggression and self-injury reliably occurred only following the occurrence of an establishing operation (a poor night's sleep for one participant, the cancelling of or delay in previous activities for the other two) *and* a discriminative stimulus (error correction or interruption by staff). They demonstrated that, following the establishing operation with an individually designed 'neutralizing routine' (a 1-hour sleep for one participant, participation in highly preferred activities for the other two) immediately led to the virtual elimination of challenging behaviour.

Changing the nature of concurrent activities

A number of studies have indicated that challenging behaviour may be substantially reduced by changing the nature or context of concurrent activities.

Curricular design and supported routines

Touchette *et al.* described the use of a scatter plot to identify the settings associated with high rates of aggression shown by a 14-year-old girl with autism and severe intellectual disabilities (Touchette *et al.*, 1985). The results of this descriptive analysis indicated that the majority of episodes of aggression were associated with certain activities, in particular her attendance at pre-vocational and community living classes. Following the re-scheduling of her weekly timetable, in which activities associated with low rates of aggression were substituted for these class activities, the girl's aggression rapidly reduced to near zero levels. They also demonstrated the rapid elimination of the serious self-injurious behaviour shown by a 23-year-old man with autism following the re-allocation of care staff. In both examples, it proved possible over time to gradually re-introduce (or fade in) the activity or person which had been associated with high rates of challenging behaviour while maintaining the treatment gains.

In an illustration of a 'molar' approach to identifying antecedent influences on challenging behaviour, Ferro *et al.* used non-participant behavioural observations to examine the association between curricular activities and challenging behaviour among 288 students with intellectual disabilities in 64 classrooms in the south eastern United States (Ferro *et al.*, 1996). Their results indicated significantly greater occurrence of challenging behaviours during activities which were non-functional, age-inappropriate or non-preferred.

Using a similar approach, several studies have reported reductions in challenging behaviour as a result of using assessments of participant preferences to design educational or vocational curricula (Cooper *et al.*, 1992; Dunlap *et al.*, 1994; Dunlap *et al.*, 1995; Dyer *et al.*, 1990; Foster-Johnson *et al.*, 1994; Vaughn and Horner, 1997). For example, Foster-Johnson *et al.* used an observational procedure to assess preference for curricular activities with three children with intellectual disabilities (Foster-Johnson *et al.*, 1994). Subsequent experimental analysis using a withdrawal design revealed higher rates of challenging behaviour during non-preferred activities and, for two of the three participants, higher rates of desirable behaviours during the preferred activities.

A small number of studies have also suggested that the actual act of choosing may be important in increasing participation (Sigafoos, 1998) and reducing challenging behaviour (Dyer *et al.*, 1990). Dunlap *et al.*, for example, attempted to untangle the effects of the act of choosing and the results of choosing (gaining access to preferred activities) in a study involving three young boys with severe emotional and behavioural difficulties (Dunlap *et al.*, 1994). They found that, when the children chose tasks, they showed greater engagement and less challenging behaviour than when simply presented with identical tasks at other times. While this obviously does not account for momentary fluctuations in preferences, it does suggest that the act of choosing itself may be important (Bannerman *et al.*, 1990; Sigafoos, 1998).

Such an approach has obvious attractions for the treatment of challenging behaviour in that: (1) it can result in rapid and marked reductions in the challenging behaviour; and (2) it may be relatively easy to sustain (if not introduce) since it requires general organizational change rather than changes in the way that carers or support staff respond to episodes of challenging behaviour. Its primary disadvantages, however, are that (1) the settings which evoke behaviour may be either important for the person's health and safety, development or quality of life (e.g. interaction with other people, requests to participate in an activity) or (2) it may be difficult to avoid the eliciting circumstances.

Environmental enrichment and non-contingent reinforcement

A number of studies have indicated that generally enriching the environment by, for example, increasing interaction with materials or introducing materials into barren environments may lead to a reduction in the rate of challenging behaviours. Thus, for example, increasing social contact (Mace and Knight, 1986), providing toys (Favell *et al.*, 1982), individually preferred activities (Lindauer *et al.*, 1999), visual stimulation (Forehand and Baumeister, 1970), leisure activities (Sigafoos and Kerr, 1994) and music (Mace *et al.*, 1989) have been associated with reduced rates of stereotypy and self-injury. Similarly, moving from materially and socially deprived institutional settings into enriched community-based residential provision is commonly associated with a reduced rate of stereotypic (although not more seriously challenging) behaviour (Emerson and Hatton, 1994; Kozma *et al.*, 2009; Walsh *et al.*, 2008).

These results are consistent with predictions made from behavioural theory. A hyperbolic relationship exists between the rate of response contingent reinforcement and behaviour (McDowell, 1982). The relationship is moderated, however, by the rate of background or response-independent reinforcement. One implication of this observation is that a particular rate of reinforcement will sustain a greater response rate in an impoverished environment than in an enriched environment. Put another way, increasing the rate of 'free' or response independent reinforcement should decrease response rate for a given rate of contingent reinforcement. Thus, the rate of behaviours maintained by positive reinforcement (external or automatic) should reduce as the background level of reinforcement increases.

As was noted earlier, however, other studies have indicated that increasing the level of stimulation in the environment through visual displays (Duker and Rasing, 1989), television (Gary et al., 1980) and crowding (McAfee, 1987) can lead to *increased* rates of stereotypy, aggression and decreased task performance. The results suggest that, for some individuals, environmental enrichment may be associated with increased rates of negative reinforcement (e.g. over-arousal, increased rates of negative peer contact). The contradictory nature of the results highlights the importance of basing interventions on prior functional assessment, since the same environmental changes may have very different effects on topographically similar behaviours.

A more specific illustration of reducing the rate of challenging behaviour by increasing the rate of background reinforcement is provided by studies of the effects of non-contingent (or response-independent) reinforcement (Carr and LeBlanc, 2006). In these studies the background rate of the *specific reinforcer maintaining the challenging behaviour* is increased, often on a fixed-time schedule. Of course, if the background rate of reinforcement is sufficiently high, it will abolish the deprivational condition, that establishes the stimulus as reinforcing and consequently eliminate challenging behaviour. That is, it should prevent maintaining stimuli acting as reinforcers in that particular context.

Mace and Lalli, for example, demonstrated that the 'delusional and hallucinatory' speech of a 46-year-old man with moderate intellectual disabilities was maintained by attention (Mace and Lalli, 1991). Subsequently, the provision of non-contingent attention on a conjunctive fixed-time, DRO schedule (reinforcer presented after a set period of time has elapsed as long as the target behaviour did not occur) resulted in the immediate reduction of bizarre speech to near zero levels. Hagopian et al. examined the effects of dense and lean schedules of non-contingent reinforcement on the attention-maintained aggressive, disruptive and self-injurious behaviour shown by four, 5-year-old identical quadruplets with intellectual disabilities and pervasive developmental disorder (Hagopian et al., 1994). They reported that: (1) the dense (FT-10 s) schedule resulted in greater reductions in disruptive behaviour (virtual elimination) than the lean (FT-5 min) schedule; (2) it was possible to gradually fade from the dense to lean schedule over a period of 55–85, 20-minute sessions while maintaining treatment gains; (3) once established on the FT-5 min schedule, it was possible to generalize treatment gains to the home setting using the children's mother as the therapist. These gains were maintained at 1- and 2-month follow-up.

Satiation involves allowing free access to the reinforcer maintaining challenging behaviour for a specified period of time. This technique has been used successfully to reduce rumination (the regurgitation and chewing of food) in people with profound intellectual disabilities (Rast et al., 1981; Rast et al., 1984). Given that the participants in these studies were underweight, increased calorific intake was in itself beneficial.

The value of approaches based on the use of non-contingent reinforcement are that: (1) they are relatively simple to implement; (2) they appear to have few side effects (Vollmer et al., 1997); and (3) they may prevent the development of deprivational conditions that set the occasion for challenging behaviour to occur. One general concern, however, is that while functionally based, such procedures are not constructional. That is, no new behaviours are established or generalized to the settings in which the person had learned a strategy for accessing particular stimuli. Indeed, the procedure results in an overall loss of opportunities for the person with severe disabilities to exert control over their environment. Given the generalized importance of our ability to exercise control (Bannerman et al., 1990), and the very limited opportunities for control available to people with severe disabilities, the use of non-contingent reinforcement on its own should be advocated with some caution.

Embedding

As was demonstrated earlier, sometimes changing relatively superficial aspects of the context in challenging behaviour occur can have a significant impact (Carr et al., 1976). Similarly, a number of studies have shown that increasing the availability of positive reinforcers or preferred materials in 'high risk' situations may significantly reduce escape-motivated challenging behaviour (Carr and Newsom, 1985; Carr et al., 1997; Kennedy, 1994a). For example, Durand and Mapstone reported substantial reductions in challenging behaviour and reduced negative affect (measured through ratings of facial expression) when 'fast-paced' music was incorporated into situations that were associated with high rates of challenging behaviour (Durand and Mapstone, 1998).

Summary

Approaches that rely on the modification of antecedent or contextual factors have a number of potential advantages. First, they can bring about rapid and significant reductions in challenging behaviour. Both the speed and magnitude of the reported changes compare well with more traditional approaches to intervention. Indeed, if the intervention is successful in removing those establishing operations that create the motivational basis for challenging behaviour, we would expect the intervention to *immediately eliminate* the challenging behaviour. To date, however, such dramatic effects have only been reported for escape-motivated challenging behaviour where preliminary descriptive or experimental analyses have been able to identify clear environmental establishing operations.

Second, approaches based on the modification of antecedent events may be relatively easy to implement and sustain over time. Such approaches place less reliance on altering the nature of carers' responses to episodes of challenging behaviour, responses which may be powerfully determined by the dynamics of the challenging behaviour itself (Taylor and Carr, 1993). Failure to sustain 'successful' intervention programmes and the re-emergence of challenging behaviour have been enduring problems faced by applied behavioural approaches.

Finally, studies to date have not reported any negative 'side effects' of interventions based on the alteration of antecedent conditions. Again, this is consistent with the underlying rationale of the approach. If the motivational bases for challenging behaviour can be removed, there is no particular reason why new challenging behaviours should emerge to replace those eliminated.

Behavioural competition and response covariation

The second set of approaches to intervention that will be examined are all based on the notion that decreases in challenging behaviour may be brought about indirectly through increasing the rate of other behaviours. Two sets of procedures which share this common aim will be discussed: the use of *functional displacement* to replace challenging behaviour with a more appropriate member of the same response class (Carr, 1988); and other procedures involving the *differential reinforcement* of other, alternative or incompatible behaviours.

Before discussing these techniques, however, some of the concepts and evidence underlying this set of approaches will be briefly reviewed. A behavioural perspective is primarily concerned with the discovery of functional relationships between behaviours, and between behaviour and environmental variables. It also views the behaviours shown by a person as the product of a dynamic system of elements, which may interact in complex and unforeseen ways. The discovery of functional relationships between behaviours led to the notion of *response classes*. These are composed of topographically distinct behaviours that have the same functional relationship to environmental events. So, for example, pressing a light switch with your thumb or index finger has the same environmental effect. As such these two behaviours are members of the same response class. Different forms of challenging behaviour may be members of the same or different response classes, and a behaviour's membership of a response class may vary over time and across settings. Intervention through functional displacement seeks to establish and/or differentially reinforce socially appropriate members of response classes containing challenging behaviour.

Other concepts have also been developed to describe the inter-relationships between behaviours, including such concepts as behavioural clusters, keystone behaviours, behavioural cusps and pivotal behaviours.

The *behavioural cluster* is a theoretically neutral term that refers to behaviours that tend to occur together in the same context. So, for example, writing an essay, drinking coffee and gazing out of the window may form a cluster of behaviours centred around the *keystone behaviour* of writing. That is, knowledge of the keystone behaviour allows us to predict the occurrence of other behaviours in the cluster. Wahler, for example, examined the correlation of 19 categories of child behaviour and six categories of social-environmental events across two settings for two boys (Wahler, 1975). He identified a number of naturally covarying behavioural clusters which were all specific to a particular setting. Clusters were, however, stable over time and across experimental phases. So, for example, the self-stimulatory behaviour of one participant was positively correlated with social contact at home, and with sustained attention to classroom work at school. He suggested that such analyses may indicate ways in which covert or low frequency behaviours may be treated indirectly and may help identify keystone behaviours whose modification may be associated with more widespread positive change.

Pivotal behaviours (Koegel and Koegel, 1988) or, more broadly, *behavioural cusps* (Rosales-Ruiz and Baer, 1997) are behaviour changes which have widespread effects by bringing the person's subsequent behaviour into contact with new contingencies and opportunities that may have far reaching consequences. Examples of pivotal behaviours include enhancing motivation and increasing responsivity to multiple cues among children with autism (Schreibman *et al.*, 1996).

Response chains are sequences of behaviour where each step in the chain is dependent upon the occurrence of the previous 'link'. Taking a bath, for example, includes a chain of behaviours (putting the plug in, running the water . . .) in which the completion of each step sets the occasion for the next step in the sequence. Performance of the complete chain is maintained by end-point reinforcing contingencies. It is possible that some examples of challenging behaviours that occur together may form response chains (Parrish and Roberts, 1993). If this were the case, then intervention focused on initial components in the chain should have generalized benefits in also preventing the occurrence of later links.

Functional displacement

Intervention through functional displacement seeks to establish and/or differentially reinforce socially appropriate members of response classes containing challenging behaviour. That is, it does not aim to alter either the antecedents that set the occasion for the behaviour to occur, or the contingencies maintaining the challenging behaviour. Rather, it seeks to introduce a new behaviour (or increase the rate of a pre-existing behaviour) that will tap into the existing contingencies and displace the challenging behaviour (Carr, 1988; Carr et al., 1994; Dyer and Larsson, 1997; O'Reilly et al., 2006).

The seminal study in this area was conducted by Carr and Durand (Carr and Durand, 1985a). First, they used experimental functional analyses to identify the processes underlying the disruptive behaviours (aggression, tantrums, self-injury, non-compliance) shown by four children with intellectual disabilities (Jim, Eve, Tom and Sue). Jim and Eve's disruptive behaviours appeared to be maintained by negative reinforcement involving escape from difficult tasks. Tom's disruptive behaviours appeared to be maintained by positive reinforcement involving teacher attention. Sue's disruptive behaviours appeared to be maintained by both negative reinforcement involving escape from difficult tasks *and* positive reinforcement involving teacher attention.

They then taught the children 'relevant' and 'irrelevant' communicative responses to the situations that elicited their challenging behaviour. The relevant response was functionally equivalent to their challenging behaviour. This involved either asking the teacher for help during difficult tasks by saying 'I don't understand' (Jim, Eve and Sue) or asking the teacher for feedback during easy tasks by asking 'Am I doing good work' (Tom and Sue). The irrelevant response was functionally unrelated to the child's challenging behaviour. This involved either asking the teacher for feedback during difficult tasks (Jim, Eve and Sue) or asking the teacher for help during easy tasks (Tom and Sue). The results of this study demonstrated immediate and dramatic reductions in each of the children's challenging behaviours when the child was taught the relevant (functionally equivalent) communicative response. Training on the irrelevant communicative response had no impact on their challenging behaviour.

Two early studies serve to illustrate the use of functional displacement to reduce challenging behaviours shown by people with more severe disabilities. Steege et al. taught two young children with severe multiple disabilities to press a microswitch that activated a tape recording to request a break from self-care activities (Steege et al., 1990). Use of this assistive device was associated with significant reductions in their escape-motivated self-injurious behaviour. Bird et al. described the use of functional communication training to eliminate the severe escape-maintained challenging behaviours of two men with severe intellectual disabilities (Gregg and Jim) (Bird et al., 1989). Gregg was taught to exchange a token for a short break from vocational tasks. Jim was taught to use the manual sign 'break'. In addition to rapid and marked reductions in challenging behaviour, spontaneous communication increased in a range of settings and, interestingly, both men spent more time on-task than they had previously and actually requested to work on tasks they had previously avoided. This suggests that one effect of the intervention was to decrease the 'aversiveness' of the negatively reinforcing tasks. This is, of course, consistent with the literature that suggests *perceived control* over potentially aversive events is an important moderator of the level of stress experienced (Bannerman *et al.*, 1990).

A number of other studies have demonstrated the viability of the procedure across a number of settings, participants and challenging behaviours and have indicated that the results may generalize across settings and therapists and be maintained over time (Carr *et al.*, 1994; Durand, 1999; Dyer and Larsson, 1997; Kurtz *et al.*, 2003). Studies have also begun to identify the conditions under which functional displacement is more or less likely to occur. Carr suggested that functional displacement is likely to occur if the replacement response is equivalent to the challenging behaviour and is also a relatively more 'efficient' response (Carr, 1988). He defined response efficiency as a complex construct reflecting the combined effects of response effort and the rate, delay and quality of reinforcement contingent upon the response. Indeed, much basic research on behavioural choice has identified these variables as predicting allocation between two concurrently available responses (Fisher and Mazur, 1997).

Horner *et al.* examined the effect of response effort on the displacement of escape-motivated aggression in a 14-year-old boy with intellectual disabilities and cerebral palsy (Horner *et al.*, 1990). They demonstrated that, while teaching an alternative response that required substantial effort (spelling out 'help please' on a personal communicator) had no impact on aggression, training in a low effort response (pressing one key to elicit the message 'help please') resulted in marked reductions in aggression and an increased use of appropriate communication. Similarly, Peck *et al.* demonstrated that variation in both duration and quality of reinforcement similarly influenced allocation of responses to trained functionally equivalent signs and challenging behaviour (Peck *et al.*, 1996).

Further support for the importance of relative response efficiency in predicting the outcomes of intervention is provided by studies that have undertaken component analyses of intervention programmes based on functional communication training. Wacker *et al.* demonstrated that the combination of functional communication training with DRO and time-out contingencies for the occurrence of challenging behaviour resulted in significantly greater reductions in challenging behaviour than functional communication training alone (Wacker *et al.*, 1990). Fisher *et al.* reported that functional communication training alone only reduced the severely challenging behaviours shown by one of three people with severe intellectual disabilities (Fisher *et al.*, 1993). However, the combination of functional communication training and punishment of the challenging behaviour (verbal reprimand plus prompting and guiding to complete five requests or 30-second physical restraint) resulted in rapid and clinically significant reductions in all challenging behaviours.

The accumulated evidence, therefore, suggests that a range of challenging behaviours may be rapidly and substantially reduced by establishing and/or differentially reinforcing a more socially appropriate member of the response class which includes the person's challenging behaviour. In addition, it would appear that the effects of intervention may persist over time and generalize to new settings. This approach is attractive in that it is functionally based, constructional and seeks to tap into contingencies of reinforcement which are known to be highly effective in maintaining behaviour over time and across settings (i.e. the contingencies maintaining challenging behaviour). The success of this approach, however, is dependent upon the alternative response being: *functionally equivalent* of the challenging behaviour; and relatively more efficient than the challenging behaviour.

The first requirement highlights the importance of conducting a thorough functional assessment prior to intervention. Indeed, it is only through such an assessment that the behavioural function of the person's challenging behaviour may be established. As was noted earlier, this may not be a simple matter, in that the processes underlying challenging behaviour may be complex and may vary over time, behaviours and across settings.

The second requirement, that the replacement response be more efficient than the challenging behaviour, has two main implications. First, in order to maximize the impact of intervention, it may be important to increase the response efficiency of the replacement behaviour *and* decrease the response efficiency of the challenging behaviour. That is, it is likely to be necessary to combine functional displacement or functional communication training with more traditional reactive strategies (e.g. extinction, time-out) to weaken the challenging behaviour. In situations in which the challenging behaviour is multiply controlled by biological and behavioural factors (e.g. self-injury maintained by extrinsic reinforcement and β-endorphin release), this may involve the combined use of behavioural and psychopharmacological treatments.

Second, evidence of the powerful effects of challenging behaviour on the performance of care staff (Taylor and Carr, 1993) suggests that it may be difficult to maintain these relative differences in response efficiency. Indeed, the behavioural account of the development of challenging behaviour through a process of shaping suggests that such behaviours may, over time, have replaced more socially appropriate functionally equivalent behaviours. Thus, the problem is often not that the person does not have more appropriate behaviours in his or her repertoire, but that environments have, over time, preferentially selected challenging behaviours. Decay in the implementation of 'successful' intervention programmes has long been a problem faced in applied settings. If such decay results in reducing the response efficiency of the alternative behaviour (e.g. care staff not attending to socially appropriate requests for breaks or attention), it is likely that the challenging behaviour will re-emerge. In many ways, teaching a functionally equivalent response to a service user may be considerably easier than ensuring that carers and care staff continue to listen to, and act upon, alternative methods of communication.

The primary disadvantages of functional displacement are, first, that its successful implementation requires skilled and intensive support during assessment and intervention. Second, it may not be appropriate in situations in which the person's challenging behaviour is maintained by either access to events which are detrimental to their health, welfare or safety (e.g. challenging behaviour maintained by sexually inappropriate contact with care staff) or, perhaps more commonly, avoidance of situations which are important to their health, welfare or quality of life (e.g. social interaction). Take, for example, the situation in which, following sexual abuse, a person with severe intellectual disabilities develops challenging behaviour to escape from physical or social contact with all carers. Would it be appropriate to simply provide the person with an alternative way of avoiding contact, or should the aim of intervention also be to help the person overcome their fear/distress of non-abusive contact?

Differential reinforcement

A more general set of approaches based on the notion of differential reinforcement also seeks to intervene indirectly on challenging behaviour by increasing the rate of other behaviours. These include: the *differential reinforcement of other* behaviour (DRO); and the *differential reinforcement of alternative* (DRA) or *incompatible* (DRI) behaviour.

The differential reinforcement of other behaviour, also known as omission training, is a non-constructional procedure involving the delivery of reinforcement contingent on the non-occurrence of the targeted challenging behaviour during an interval of time or, more unusually, at a specific point in time (momentary DRO). Under a DRO schedule, the nature of the 'other' behaviours are not specified. Reinforcement is provided as long as the challenging behaviour does not occur. In effect, a DRO schedule is equivalent to time-out from a newly imposed contingency of positive reinforcement (Rolider and Van Houten, 1990).

The differential reinforcement of alternative or incompatible behaviour involves the delivery of reinforcement contingent on the occurrence of a specified alternative behaviour (DRA) or a behaviour that is physically incompatible with the challenging behaviour (DRI). Functional displacement is, in effect, a particular form of DRA in which the reinforcing contingency is identical to that maintaining the challenging behaviour.

Individual studies have reported marked variability in the outcomes associated with differential reinforcement procedures, with results ranging from complete suppression, through marginal improvements to increases in the rate of challenging behaviour over baseline (Carr *et al.*, 1990b; Pretscher *et al.*, 2009). In general, however, it would appear that such procedures may not be particularly effective in reducing severely challenging behaviours (Carr *et al.*, 1990b; Didden *et al.*, 1997; Harvey *et al.*, 2009; Scotti *et al.*, 1991b; Whitaker, 1993).

As has been discussed above, studies of behavioural choice suggest that a person's allocation of time between concurrently available alternatives (e.g. attending to a task, engaging in self-injurious behaviour, gazing out of the window) is a function of response effort and the rate, quality and immediacy of reinforcement. As such, these factors should predict the effectiveness of differential reinforcement procedures as well as functional displacement. Thus, an effective procedure should aim to ensure that:

- the alternative behaviour requires less effort than the person's challenging behaviour;
- the rate of reinforcement delivered contingent on the alternative behaviour is greater than the rate of reinforcement maintaining the challenging behaviour;
- reinforcement is delivered immediately upon occurrence of the alternative behaviour;
- the reinforcers selected are more powerful than those maintaining the challenging behaviour, preferably through the use of empirical procedures to identify reinforcer selection.

The effectiveness of differential reinforcement procedures may also be enhanced by selecting alternative behaviours that show a natural negative covariation with the targeted challenging behaviour. Parrish *et al.*, for example, demonstrated the natural negative covariation of compliance and challenging behaviours, including aggression, property destruction, pica and disruption, among four children with intellectual disabilities (Parrish *et al.*, 1986). As compliance increased, due to the effects of either differential reinforcement or guided compliance, challenging behaviours decreased. These suggestions for improving the effectiveness of differential reinforcement procedures again highlight the importance of preceding intervention with a thorough functional assessment.

Such procedures are relatively simple to administer in that they do not require skilled performance from care staff. The main drawbacks of these procedures, however, are that reinforcer satiation may occur at brief inter-reinforcement intervals, their implementation requires intensive monitoring of user behaviour and questionable efficacy.

Modification of maintaining contingencies: extinction

The approaches discussed so far have not involved any *direct* alteration of the contingencies maintaining the person's challenging behaviour. Antecedent manipulations and differential reinforcement may both, of course, indirectly influence the power of the maintaining contingencies through modifying establishing operations, by increasing the rate of 'free' reinforcement or re-inforcement available for competing behaviours. Extinction procedures involve the direct modification of the contingencies responsible for maintaining the challenging behaviour.

Specifically, extinction procedures involve ensuring that the contingencies responsible for maintaining the person's challenging behaviour are no longer operative. Thus, for example, if functional assessment has indicated that an individual's aggression is maintained by positive social reinforcement involving attention from care staff, an extinction procedure would ensure that such positive reinforcers were no longer delivered contingent upon the person's challenging behaviour.

Lovaas and Simmons, for example, used an extinction procedure to reduce the attention-maintained severe self-injurious behaviour shown by two boys with severe intellectual disabilities (Lovaas and Simmons, 1969). The procedure involved leaving each boy alone in an observation room for 90-minute sessions. Within eight sessions (12 hours), John's self-injury had been eliminated. Prior to this, however, he had hit himself 9000 times during the extinction sessions. Gregg's self-injury took much longer to extinguish. These effects were, however, situationally specific, in that treatment gains failed to generalize to other settings.

Escape extinction involves ensuring that negative reinforcers are not with-drawn contingent upon the person's challenging behaviour (e.g. preventing escape from an aversive situation contingent upon challenging behaviour). Such procedures have been used to successfully reduce escape-maintained challenging behaviour (Iwata *et al.*, 1994a).

Sensory extinction procedures involve attempting to block the sensory or perceptual feedback from challenging behaviours maintained by automatic reinforcement (Rincover and Devany, 1982). Such procedures have been employed to reduce self-injurious and stereotypic behaviours apparently main-tained by automatic reinforcement (Rincover and Devany, 1982).

While extinction may be effective, its use does have a number of significant problems. First, the rate, intensity and variability of challenging behaviour are likely to increase in a significant minority of cases during the initial stages of an extinction programme (Lerman and Iwata, 1995). Such *extinction bursts* may place the physical safety of the person in jeopardy and are likely to be distressing to carers and care staff. Second, extinction procedures may need to be imple-mented with a high degree of consistency. Otherwise, the procedure would be equivalent to simply reducing the rate of reinforcement for the person's challenging behaviour. While this may have the effect of reducing response rate (see above), it may not bring about socially or clinically significant improve-ment. Third, as noted above, the effects of extinction procedures may not generalize to new situations. Finally, as a non-constructional approach, extinction may be associated with unwanted changes in collateral behaviours. Given the problems associated with extinction procedures, it is highly unlikely that they would be implemented on their own. They are often, however, included as an important component in complex treatment packages.

Default technologies: punishment

There are two types of contingent relationship between behaviour and re-inforcers that are sometimes important in directly *reducing or eliminating* operant behaviour. *Positive punishment* refers to a decrease in the rate of a behaviour as a result of the contingent *presentation* of a (negatively) reinforcing stimulus (positive punisher). Illustrative examples of positive punishment include the use by parents of reprimands to reduce the unruly behaviour of their children. *Negative punishment* refers to a decrease in the rate of a behaviour as a result of the contingent *withdrawal* of a (positively) reinforcing stimulus (negative punisher). Examples of negative punishment include the use of fines to prevent inappropriate parking (negative punisher: loss of money) and the with-drawal of attention to reduce the overbearing or rude behaviour of colleagues.

Over the past three decades, numerous studies have demonstrated that punishment procedures can produce significant reductions in severe challen-ging behaviours shown by people with severe intellectual disabilities. Indeed, meta-analyses of the intervention literature indicate that extinction and punishment-based procedures are the most effective approaches available, both immediately and at follow-up, if the goal is to eliminate challenging behaviour (Didden *et al.*, 1997; Scotti *et al.*, 1991b).

The use of punishment-based procedures is, however, deeply problematic as the procedures (if not the outcomes) are nowadays considered to be socially unacceptable. This has led to a situation in which punishment procedures may be best viewed as 'default technologies' (Iwata, 1988). That is, approaches that should only be considered when: (a) alternative approaches have failed or are not feasible; (b) the costs of not intervening outweigh the costs and risks associated with the use of such procedures; (c) all appropriate consent proce-dures have been followed. In the sections below, some of the approaches to punishment that have been successfully used to reduce severely challenging behaviours will be briefly reviewed.

Response cost: time-out and visual screening

Response cost (or negative punishment) refers to the reduction in the rate of a behaviour resulting from the *withdrawal* of positive reinforcers contingent upon its occurrence. *Time-out* is a clinical procedure in which opportunity for positive reinforcement is removed or reduced for a set period following the occurrence of a target behaviour. This may involve the brief seclusion of the person in a barren environment, removal to a less stimulating part of the current setting or the withdrawal of potentially positively reinforcing activities or events from the vicinity of the person.

Time-out has been shown to be successful in reducing challenging behaviours shown by people with severe intellectual disabilities (Cataldo, 1991). However, 'time-out' may also lead to an increase in the rate of escape-motivated challenging behaviour (Durand et al., 1989; Solnick et al., 1977). For such behaviours, the implementation of a typical exclusionary time-out procedure is likely to negatively reinforce the targeted behaviour. Research conducted on the parameters of time-out have suggested that short durations are as effective as long durations, the use of contingent delay for release from time-out (i.e. release is delayed until challenging behaviours have stopped) may be unnecessary and the effectiveness of the procedure may be enhanced by combining time-out with differential reinforcement of more appropriate behaviour. While potentially effective, the implementation of time-out and response-cost procedures may themselves set the occasion for the occurrence of challenging behaviour as the person seeks to avoid or escape from the punishing contingency.

Visual or *facial screening* involves the brief (5–15 seconds) blocking of vision contingent upon the occurrence of challenging behaviour, a procedure that has been shown to bring about rapid, significant and, at times, persistent reductions in self-injurious behaviour, screaming and stereotypy (Rojahn and Marshburn, 1992). Similarly with the use of time-out, visual screening may set the occasion for the occurrence of challenging behaviour as the person seeks to avoid or escape from the punishing contingency (Rojahn & Marshburn, 1992).

Positive punishment

Positive punishment refers to the reduction in the rate of a behaviour as a result of the contingent presentation of a punishing stimulus. A wide range of punishing stimuli have been employed to reduce challenging behaviour. Apart from verbal reprimands, all approaches have been shown to be effective in some instances in bringing about short- and medium-term reductions in severe challenging behaviour (Cataldo, 1991).

Azrin et al., for example, demonstrated that the combination of the differential reinforcement of incompatible behaviour (DRI), response interruption and contingent manual restraint for a 2-minute period brought about rapid and significant reductions in the severe long-standing self-injurious behaviour shown by one girl, two women and six men with severe intellectual disabilities. Across all participants, self-injury was reduced to 11% of baseline levels (Azrin et al., 1988).

The use of punishment-based procedures raises a number of issues. Several commentators have suggested that the use of punishment may be associated with unacceptably high rates of negative 'side effects' (Guess et al., 1987).

Indeed, negative outcomes associated with the use of punishment have included increases in non-targeted challenging behaviour, increased incontinence and decreased appetite (Cataldo, 1991). However, reviews of applied research have consistently noted that: (a) reporting of side effects is often anecdotal, and (b) the reporting of positive side effects (e.g. increased sociability, increased responsiveness, reduced medication, reduced use of restraints) consistently outweighs the reporting of negative side effects in the applied literature (Cataldo, 1991). Nevertheless, as with procedures based on negative punishment, the implementation of punishment-based procedures may set the occasion for the occurrence of challenging behaviour as the person seeks to avoid or escape from the punishing contingency (Linscheid, 1992). In addition, problems may be encountered in the maintenance of treatment gains, especially over the longer term.

Cognitive-behavioural approaches, self-management and self-control

Over the last decade there has been a growing interest in the use of cognitive behavioural approaches and the use of self-management or self-control procedures by people with intellectual disabilities. Studies involving people with mild or moderate intellectual disabilities have indicated that: (1) people can reliably self-report on internal states and cognitions; (2) self-monitoring alone may reduce self-injury, aggressive and stereotypic behaviour; (3) more complex self-management procedures including anger management training and social problem-solving skills may reduce aggressive, disruptive, stereotypic and self-injurious behaviour (Dagnan et al., 2007; Kroese et al., 1997). However, the applicability of such procedures to people with more severe disabilities is unclear. Of particular importance is the relationship between the development of language and the emergence of rule-governed behaviour, of which self-management or self-regulation is an example.

However, the results of studies investigating self-management among young children with autism suggest that such approaches may be more applicable to people with severe disabilities than is commonly thought. For example, Koegel and Koegel investigated the applicability of self-management procedures in the reduction of stereotypic behaviours shown by four children with autism (Koegel and Koegel, 1990). The children's mental ages ranged from 2 years 9 months to 5 years 11 months. Their chronological age ranged from 9 to 14 years. Each child displayed between three and six distinct forms of stereotypic behaviour. Implementation of an externally reinforced self-monitoring procedures was associated with highly significant reductions in stereotypy for three of the children. The fourth child, who had the highest mental age, showed consistent but less pronounced reductions in stereotypy.

Multi-component strategies

Much of the research literature has been concerned with determining the efficacy of discrete approaches to intervention. In clinical practice, however, the need to bring about rapid and significant change argues for the use of complex multi-component intervention strategies (Cameron *et al.*, 1998; Carr *et al.*, 1994; Ricciardi, 2006; Risley, 1996). Carr and Carlson, for example, employed a complex package involving choice, embedding, functional communication training, building tolerance for delay of reinforcement and the presentation of discriminative stimuli for non-problem behaviours to teach shopping skills to three adolescent boys with autism and severe intellectual disabilities (Carr and Carlson, 1993). Following the implementation of the programme all participants were able to shop in supermarkets and displayed virtually no challenging behaviour during this activity. Similarly, Saunders introduced the idea of addressing challenging behaviour through the establishment of *supported routines* (Saunders and Saunders, 1998). This fundamentally constructional approach involves the development of detailed procedures for the 'comprehensive enablement' of competent performance in situations which may elicit challenging behaviour.

Summary

Table 11.1 summarizes some of the main advantages and disadvantages of the approaches to intervention discussed in this chapter. The evidence that has been reviewed in earlier chapters indicated that severely challenging behaviours may be highly persistent.

To recapitulate:

- adults who come to the attention of specialized services have commonly shown the same challenging behaviours for a decade or more;
- the vast majority of people who show self-injurious behaviour at one point in time, are also likely to do so many years later;
- longer-term follow up of 'successful' intervention programmes often report a very high rate of relapse or, alternatively, indicate that challenging behaviours tend to persist, but at a much lower intensity and/or rate.

Attention was also drawn to some of the personal and social consequences which the person may experience as a result of his or her challenging behaviour. These include: physical injury, ill health and the development of secondary sensory or neurological impairments; abuse; inappropriate treatment involving the long-term prescription of neuroleptics; the use of mechanical restraints and protective devices; exposure to unnecessarily degrading or abusive psychological treatments; exclusion from community settings, relationships and services; social and material deprivation and systematic neglect.

Table 11.1. Summary of behavioural approaches to intervention

Approach	Constructional?	Functional?	Primary advantages	Primary disadvantages
Modification of biobehavioural state				
Modification of idiosyncratic establishing operations	No	Yes	Immediate and significant reductions in challenging behaviour possible ease of implementation	Requires detailed functional assessment
Changing the nature of preceding activities				
Modify idiosyncratic setting events	No	Yes	Immediate and significant reductions in challenging behaviour possible ease of implementation	Requires detailed functional assessment
Non-contingent exercise	No	No	Ease of implementation broad-based effects possible positive collateral changes (e.g. sleeping, general health benefits) possible when maintaining factors unknown	May be ineffective for, or increase, some escape-motivated challenging behaviour temporary effects
Interspersed requests (behavioural momentum)	No	Yes	Immediate and significant reductions in challenging behaviour ease of implementation	Requires detailed functional assessment
Neutralizing routines	No	Yes	Immediate and significant reductions in challenging behaviour possible ease of implementation	Requires detailed functional assessment

Table 11.1. (cont.)

Approach	Constructional?	Functional?	Primary advantages	Primary disadvantages
Changing the nature of concurrent activities: curricular design and supported routines				
Schedule activities to avoid antecedents or on basis of preferences	No	Yes	Immediate and significant reductions in challenging behaviour ease of implementation	May not be feasible to avoid antecedents: antecedents may be important for health or welfare of person requires detailed functional assessment
Increase task variety	No	Yes	Immediate and significant reductions in challenging behaviour ease of implementation	Requires detailed functional assessment
Increase opportunities for choice making	No	No	Possible broad-based effects possible positive collateral changes (e.g. reduced stress) possible when maintaining factors unknown	Unknown effectiveness may be complex to implement
Stimulus fading	No	Yes	May help reduce escape-motivated challenging behaviour elicited by conditioned arousal may help re-introduce antecedents important to health/welfare of person	May not be feasible to control access to antecedents relatively slow acting requires detailed functional assessment

Modify idiosyncratic setting events	No	Yes	Immediate and significant reductions in challenging behaviour possible ease of implementation	Requires detailed functional assessment

Changing the nature of concurrent activities: environmental enrichment and non-contingent reinforcement

Increase level of background stimulation	No	No	Simple to sustain ease of implementation broad-based effects possible positive collateral changes (e.g. wakefulness) possible when maintaining factors unknown	May be ineffective for or increase escape-motivated challenging behaviours may be difficult to implement initially
Non-contingent reinforcement and satiation	No	Yes	Immediate and significant reductions in challenging behaviour	Requires detailed functional assessment

Embedding

Modify idiosyncratic setting events	No	Yes	Immediate and significant reductions in challenging behaviour possible ease of implementation	Requires detailed functional assessment

Response covariation

Functional displacement	Yes	Yes	Immediate and significant reductions in challenging behaviour	Requires detailed functional assessment complex implementation May involve avoidance of activities important for health/welfare of person

Table 11.1. (cont.)

Approach	Constructional?	Functional?	Primary advantages	Primary disadvantages
Differential reinforcement of other behaviour (DRO)	No	No	Possible when maintaining factors unknown	Complex or intensive implementation
Differential reinforcement of incompatible (DRI) or alternative (DRA) behaviour	Yes	?	Possible when maintaining factors unknown	Complex or intensive implementation
Supported routines	Yes	Yes	Immediate and significant reductions in challenging behaviour highly constructional	Requires detailed functional assessment possibly complex or intensive implementation
Modification of maintaining contingencies				
Extinction	No	Yes		Requires detailed functional assessment complex or intensive implementation temporary increases in rate/variety/intensity of challenging behaviour slow acting poor generalization low procedural acceptability
Punishment (default technologies)				
Time-out	No	No		Requires detailed functional assessment complex or

Visual screening	No	No	Possible when maintaining factors unknown Immediate and significant reductions in challenging behaviour	intensive implementation poor generalization low procedural acceptability Complex or intensive implementation Possibly poor generalization low procedural acceptability
Positive punishment	No	No	Possible when maintaining factors unknown and significant reductions in challenging behaviour	Complex or intensive implementation possibly poor generalization low procedural acceptability

In the light of these observations, it is important to attempt to determine the general effectiveness of behavioural approaches in bringing about socially significant and durable change. Two aspects of the nature of the available evidence militate against being able to provide a clear answer to this important question.

First, a reliance in the research literature on single-subject experimental designs, when combined with the tendency not to report treatment failures, does mean that we know little about the extent to which the results of successful interventions may be generalized across individuals, therapists and settings. Thus, while single-subject designs often have a very high internal validity (i.e. they demonstrate that the observed changes are due to a particular intervention), systematic replication is required to determine whether the same results can be obtained with other participants, other therapists and in other settings. Unfortunately, such *systematic* replication is extremely rare in this field. As a result, while we are able to conclude that various behavioural procedures *can* bring about significant change, we cannot predict with any confidence the proportion of 'cases' in which this is likely to be achieved. Similarly, reliance on single-subject designs means that there is only limited knowledge with regards to the characteristics of the behaviour, participants or setting that are likely to influence the impact of an intervention.

The second major limitation in the available evidence concerns restrictions on the range of outcomes evaluated, aspects of response and stimulus generalization and the length of time over which the durability of intervention gains are assessed. The failure to assess the maintenance or durability of treatment effects is highlighted by the observation that, of the 366 outcomes from 109 studies of positive behavioural support reviewed by Carr *et al.*, information on maintenance over a period of more than 1 year was available for only seven (2%) of outcomes (Carr *et al.*, 1999; Dunlap *et al.*, 1999; Scotti *et al.*, 1996).

This means that relatively little is known regarding such factors as: collateral changes or the 'side effects' of intervention: the contextual control of challenging behaviour and the generalization of the effects of intervention to new settings, behaviours and people; the long-term outcomes of intervention; and the broader social validity of intervention when applied in community-based settings. Nevertheless, the accumulated evidence does indicate that behavioural approaches *can* be effective in bringing about rapid, significant and widespread reductions in severely challenging behaviours and that such changes *may* be associated with a range of positive 'side effects', *may* generalize to new settings, and *may* be maintained over long periods of time (Campbell, 2003; Carr *et al.*, 1999; Didden *et al.*, 1997; Harvey *et al.*, 2009; Marquis *et al.*, 2000; Scotti *et al.*, 1991b).

The situational management of challenging behaviour

David Allen

Associate Clinical Director, Directorate of Learning Disability Services,
ABMUHB and Professor of Clinical Psychology in Learning Disability,
Cardiff University, Cardiff, Wales.

So far, this book has been primarily concerned with proactive interventions designed to help change challenging behaviour. This chapter describes key issues and considerations in relation to the management of such behaviour when it occurs. It proposes that situational management strategies are a necessary component of comprehensive intervention for many individuals with intellectual disabilities and challenging behaviour. The characteristics of these strategies and data on their usage and effectiveness will be outlined. Based on the latter, current deficiencies in establishing the social validity of situational strategies will be identified and requirements for addressing these deficiencies discussed.

The need for behaviour management strategies

A defining characteristic of challenging behaviours is that they pose risks either to the person displaying them or to those people who provide their care and support. As described in earlier chapters, these behaviours can result in serious physical harm (Allen et al., 2006; Allen, 2008; Jones et al., 2007; Konarski et al., 1997); they can also result in significant emotional harm (Bromley and Emerson, 1995; Cambridge, 1999; Cottle et al., 1995; Jenkins et al., 1997; Lundstrom et al., 2007; Qureshi, 1990; Rowett and Breakwell, 1992).

Applied correctly, the constructive behavioural intervention measures described elsewhere in this book can clearly bring great benefits to many individuals with intellectual disabilities and their carers. Though differing slightly in their emphasis and outcomes, independent meta-analyses offer repeated confirmation of this fact (Ball et al., 2004; Campbell, 2003; Carr et al., 1999; Didden et al., 1997; Didden et al., 2006; Harvey et al., 2009; Marquis et al., 2000; Scotti et al., 1991b; Scotti et al., 1996; Whitaker, 1993). These same meta-analyses also indicate that there are limitations to these approaches which have important practical and clinical implications. These include the

Challenging Behaviour, 3rd edn, ed. Eric Emerson and Stewart L. Einfeld. Published by Cambridge University Press. © E. Emerson and S. L. Einfeld 2011.

fact that, even with successful interventions that are carried out under relatively well-controlled conditions, the complete elimination of challenging behaviour from individual repertoires is hard to achieve (Didden *et al.*, 1997; Scotti *et al.*, 1991b; Whitaker, 1993). Furthermore, success rates may be lower with outwardly directed behaviours (such as physical aggression towards others) than with more inwardly directed behaviours (such as self-injury) (Didden *et al.*, 1997; Scotti *et al.*, 1991b). Interventions are less effective with lower frequency behaviours, which is problematic if these are also high intensity behaviours (Whitaker, 1993). Also, much of the earlier behavioural intervention literature focused on less severe forms of challenging behaviour (which were therefore likely to pose fewer risks) (Carr *et al.*, 1999). Of particular significance is the fact that most constructive interventions (particularly those that involve skill-building either for the person with intellectual disability or their carers) will take time to become established, meaning that risk behaviours will continue to be displayed in the interim.

These considerations highlight the need to incorporate recommendations for the situational management of challenging behaviours alongside constructive interventions for behaviour change within behavioural support plans if such plans are to be truly comprehensive. Situational management involves giving clear guidance as to how to respond when challenging behaviours occur. The term 'reactive strategies' is another commonly used descriptor for such interventions (LaVigna *et al.*, 1989).

Failing to address situational management has a number of possible consequences. Most obviously, service users and their carers will continue to be at risk of getting hurt when challenging behaviours occur. A secondary consequence is that the latter may be more reluctant to implement constructive behaviour change strategies with someone of whom they are fearful. As described below, in the absence of the prescription of recommended strategies for responding to behaviour, carers will also tend to construct their own informal responses. Although well intended, such improvised approaches often have the potential to significantly increase risk. It may also be the case that failing to clearly prescribe appropriate standards, or prescribing the wrong standards, for situational management may contribute to the physical and emotional abuse of people with intellectual disabilities and challenging behaviour (Baker and Allen, 2001) and also to increased injuries and compensation claims from care staff (Bowie, 1996; National Taskforce on Violence Against Social Care Staff, 2000).

The characteristics of situational management strategies

Situational management strategies have been noted to have the following characteristics (Allen *et al.*, 2005; Carr *et al.*, 1994; LaVigna *et al.*, 1989).

- Situational behaviour management strategies are not in themselves 'treatments' – they are not constructive and not concerned with altering challenging behaviour in the long term.
- Their only aim is to achieve safe and rapid control over risk behaviours in the short term.
- As such, they provide as a 'window of opportunity' through which more proactive behaviour change interventions can be delivered.

These points serve to further emphasize the point that situational management plays a limited, albeit often critically important, role in the support of people who have challenging behaviour.

A typology of situational behaviour management strategies

Challenging behaviours present varying levels of risk and therefore merit varying levels of response; as behaviour is dynamic, levels of risk and therefore levels of required response may also need to vary within a specific incident. Reflecting this fact, situational management responses can be classified into two basic types: non-physical and physical (see Table 12.1 below).

Clearly, non-physical situational management strategies are less intrusive and less risky than physical ones. Within the range of available physical strategies, the use of personal space is the least intrusive option, followed by evasive techniques and the use of restraint and medication. No exact categorization of intrusiveness is possible, however, and the position of any strategy in a hierarchy is, to some extent, dependent upon the perception of the person in receipt of it. As an example, many people would probably feel that brief restraint is less aversive than seclusion, but for someone with autism who is socially avoidant, seclusion may be a relatively non-aversive (and possibly reinforcing strategy), while the use of restraint may be highly aversive (Blackburn, 2006). To add further complexity, some interventions (e.g. the administration of rapid tranquillization or placing someone in seclusion) almost always involve the use of other strategies (typically restraint) in order for them to be implemented; it is therefore hard to rate the intrusiveness of individual strategies when they may be used almost always in combination with others.

Over the last two decades, considerable attention has been paid to debating how the inherently aversive nature of some physical situational management strategies could be reduced. In relation to the use of self-protective and personal restraint within the United Kingdom, this attention has focused in the main on the rejection of procedures designed to deliberately inflict pain on the person displaying challenging behaviour for their effectiveness and on the use of prone (i.e. face down on the floor) restraint. As documented elsewhere (Allen and Harris, 2000), pain compliance procedures were originally designed for use in the UK prison service but then introduced into a wide

Table 12.1. Types of situational management

Category of intervention	Specific strategies	Examples
Non-physical	Active listening	'Listening' for early behavioural indicators (e.g. increased or decreased verbalization, pacing, etc.) that challenging behaviour may be imminent (LaVigna and Willis, 2002) and then intervening early to diffuse them
	Stimulus change or removal	Early intervention may involve 'switching off' known provocative environmental or interpersonal triggers for challenging behaviour or introducing a novel stimulus that may have a distracting value (LaVigna and Willis, 1994)
	Modifying Kinesic (non-verbal) communication	Modifying eye contact, body posture and position in order to minimize threat (Bowie, 1996)
	Modifying verbal communication	Avoiding the use of provocative expressions or threats of consequences; employing calm, low tones; keeping communications clear and brief so as to reduce misunderstanding (Bowie, 1996)
	Employ relaxation and coping skills	Prompting challenging individuals to use relaxation (Cautela and Groden, 1978) or cognitive behavioural coping skills previously learnt via anger management training, etc. (Black *et al.*, 1997).
	Don't ignore behaviour (under specific conditions)	Attention motivated behaviours should not be ignored as this risks behavioural escalation (LaVigna and Willis, 2002)
	Diversion to a reinforcing or compelling event	Introduction of a highly reinforcing activity or diversion to a compulsive activity that the individual feels compelled to do (LaVigna and Willis, 2002)
	Strategic capitulation	Providing the person with the known reinforcer for their behaviour early on in a behavioural episode in order to prevent further escalation (has to be coupled with high-rate access to the reinforcer at times on non-crisis) (LaVigna and Willis, 2002)
	Avoid natural consequences	Natural consequences that may have an aversive component for the challenging person in order to reduce possible escalation (LaVigna and Willis, 2002)
	Avoid punishing	The delivery of punishment runs the risk 'fight' rather than 'flight' reactions and should generally be avoided in crisis scenarios (LaVigna and Willis, 2002)

Physical	Proxemics	Increasing the personal space between challenging individuals and carers in order to reduce threat levels and increase carer safety (Bowie, 1996)
	Using touch	Using touch to reassure fearful service users (Bowie, 1996) [1]
	Self-protective procedures	The use of physical 'breakaway' techniques by carers to escape from grabs or holds applied by challenging individuals (Rogers et al., 2006; Wright et al., 2005)
	Personal Restraint	The application of force to present movement by one or more carers holding the challenging individual, typically in the form of basket holds (whereby a person's hands are secured in an 'X' pattern across their chest by a carer standing or kneeling behind them), supine (face up whilst held on the floor), prone (face down whilst held on the floor) or seated restraint (McDonnell et al., 1991; Wright et al., 2005)
	Environmental Restraint	The locking of doors, etc. to prevent egress either via formal seclusion or more informal means (Mental Health Act Commission, 2006)
	Mechanical Restraint	The use of splints, belts and ties to restrict the movement of individual limbs or to completely immobilize the challenging individual (Jones et al., 2007;NYS Commission on Quality of Care for the Mentally Disabled, 1994)
Chemical	Medication	The use of psychotropic medication via as required or regular doses of medication in order to achieve levels of sedation that preclude major challenging behaviours occurring (National Institute for Clinical Excellence, 2005)

[1] A strategy only for use in early behavioural escalation and a potentially high-risk one in that touch may be perceived as threatening, especially with people who have a history of being subjected to intrusive physical interventions.

variety of care settings for a wide variety of different service user groups in an essentially undiluted fashion. Not surprisingly, good practice guidelines (British Institute of Learning Disabilities, 2006; Harris *et al.*, 2008; Royal College of Psychiatrists, 1995) subsequently railed against the use of such procedures with people who have intellectual disabilities, some of whom may have elevated pain thresholds (Biersdorff, 1991, 1994; Symons *et al.*, 2008), and may therefore require an extreme application of such procedures before pain-compliance responses are elicited. Interestingly, policy statements have tended to adopt a more equivocal approach which apparently allows for the use of such procedures if necessary (Department of Health & Department for Education and Skills, 2002; Harris *et al.*, 2008; Welsh Assembly Government, 2005).

The use of prone restraint is contentious because of its being implicated in a substantial number of fatalities during restraint (Nunno *et al.*, 2006; Paterson *et al.*, 2003; Weiss, 1998). Although definitive evidence is lacking (Lancaster *et al.*, 2008; Mohr *et al.*, 2003; Parkes and Carson, 2008; Whittington *et al.*, 2006), while prone restraint is probably the position of greatest risk in terms of service user health, it is neither a necessary or sufficient condition to cause death. Risks increase significantly if certain additional physical interventions (notably, immobilization of the person's hands behind their back; obstruction of the airways; the application of additional pressure to the back, neck or trunk; or pressure on the carotid or vagus nerve) are employed during prone restraint and/or the person being restrained has pre-existing health problems (especially cardio-vascular problems). It has been argued that, given their poor general health profile overall, people with intellectual disabilities may constitute a particular frail group in terms of prone restraint use (Allen, 2008). Such are the concerns about this type of restraint that its use has been proscribed in some countries (Welsh Assembly Government, 2005) and North American states (Bullard *et al.*, 2003).

The debate on the use of such controversial situational management strategies has in many ways mirrored that on default behaviour change strategies described in Chapter 11. As with the 'aversives debate' on behaviour change strategies, the resulting controversy has also stimulated the development of alternative intervention approaches, which in this case reject the use of pain compliance, prone restraint and other intrusive physical interventions in an attempt to achieve more humane and ethical behaviour management (Allen *et al.*, 1997; McDonnell and Sturmey, 2000). Similar debates have taken place around the use of seclusion and concerns expressed that seclusion 'by another name' (e.g. 'therapeutic isolation', 'removal to a "calming room"', 'de-escalation rooms') (Mental Health Act Commission, 2006) seems common-place in many services. Some authorities (Masters, 2008) have argued cogently for the continued use of dedicated environments where challenging individuals can be helped to calm, but stressed that the modernization of 'seclusion' requires that the spaces concerned need to be made highly attractive (e.g. via the use of mood lighting and appropriate music) as opposed to unpleasant and barren. Masters also argues that the more attractive such calming spaces are, the less likely it is that restraint will be necessary to place individuals in them; however, in barren or un-stimulating care environments, such humanizing initiatives also run the risk of creating highly reinforcing settings, the use of which might inadvertently increase rates of challenging behaviour.

Epidemiology

How frequently are situational management strategies employed with people who have intellectual disabilities? Emerson reported the use of restraint for 28%–67% of children and 8%–57% of adults with intellectual disability and challenging behaviour, based on the analysis of data from a series of epidemiological studies (Emerson, 2002). The equivalent figures for seclusion were 32%–68% and 15%–39%, and 1%–6% and 15%–35% for emergency sedation. Others have reported similarly high rates of use (Deveau and McGill, 2009; Lowe et al., 2005; Robertson et al., 2005; Sturmey, 2009). Given that many services for people with intellectual disabilities often use informal interventions (i.e. ones that have not been sanctioned by appropriate professionals or documented in formal care plans), it is possible that these figures actually underestimate the use of situational management strategies. This is supported by research conducted by Feldman and colleagues, in which interview methods were used to identify formal and informal interventions used in services in Ontario, Canada (Feldman et al., 2004). A total of over 2500 interventions were identified, and 26.9% of these were concerned with situational management. Of the latter, 63% were informal, and 43% of these were assessed as being dangerous.

Limited but comparable data exist regarding the use of situational management in family settings. Adams and Allen reported that parental physical intervention was the most common response to aggressive behaviour in 56% of children referred to a specialist behavioural intervention team (Adams and Allen, 2001), while a national survey (Allen et al., 2006) found that 88% of parents reported using physical intervention with their children at some point and that 21% did so frequently. Personal restraint was most common in the latter study, but mechanical and environmental restraints were also reported. Only 25% of parents had received training in situational management and many of the physical interventions used had therefore been improvised and were extremely dangerous (e.g. using prone restraint, applying weight to the back of the restrained child, and headlocks).

A number of studies have attempted to identify risk factors for the use of situational management strategies. Emerson (2002) found that severity of intellectual impairment/ adaptive behaviour; the presence of communicative difficulties; age (younger age in adults with restraint, older age in children with seclusion); male gender, ethnicity; and diagnoses of autism or mental health problems were predictive of situational management use. Attending a special school, living in residential care, not attending a day service, living in a residence with less normal architectural features, higher staffing levels and service user numbers were identified as environmental risk factors. Allen *et al.* found that restraint use was predicted by the presence of destructive behaviour, having behavioural plans in place for specific forms of challenging behaviour, detention under mental health legislation and lower levels of adaptive behaviour; seclusion use by having more severe challenging behaviour, the presence of destructive behaviour and being placed in a service away from the person's area of origin; and sedation by detention under mental health legislation and having behavioural plans in place for specific forms of challenging behaviour (Allen *et al.*, 2009). In addition, younger participants were more likely to be restrained and older participants to receive emergency medication, a finding that was presumably indicative of the problems inherent in applying physical interventions to larger, stronger people. Those individuals who were restrained were also likely to experience both seclusion and sedation. McGill *et al.* found that individuals who experienced restraint, seclusion or emergency medication were more likely to be male, young, not subject to legal detention, and to be described as having autistic spectrum disorder (McGill *et al.*, 2009) . However, Sturmey found only limited evidence that between-participant differences in challenging behaviour were predictive of restraint use within two institutional samples (Sturmey, 1999; Sturmey *et al.*, 2005).

Mason, in a study conducted within a special hospital for individuals with very high-risk behaviours and forensic needs, reported that individuals with intellectual disability tended to be secluded more frequently than individuals without, but that the behaviours leading to seclusion did not appear to warrant this action and that the individuals concerned responded badly to this form of intervention (Mason, 1996). Another hospital study by Rangecroft and Colleagues found that many of those secluded had severe intellectual disability, high rates of epilepsy and long histories of institutionalization (Rangecroft *et al.*, 1997).

Two studies have attempted to explore whether staff attributions for behaviour impact on situational management techniques selected. In a retrospective analysis of record sheets for incidents of restraint, seclusion and emergency medication use, Leggett and Silvester found that the use of seclusion was associated with controllable service user attributions (i.e. the person could have done something to avoid the incident if they wished) and uncontrollable staff attributions (i.e. it is unlikely that the staff member could have done anything to alter the course of the incident) (Leggett and Silvester, 2003). The use of emergency medication was associated with uncontrollable service user attributions, but only with males. Dagnan and Weston found that there was no association between attributional measures and situational management options chosen, but that physical intervention was much more likely to be used in response to physical rather than verbal aggression (Dagnan and Weston, 2006).

Given the established imbalance between the number of people with intellectual disabilities who are in receipt of constructive behaviour change strategies (Harris and Russell, 1998; Lowe *et al.*, 2005; Oliver *et al.*, 1987; Qureshi, 1994) and the numbers who appear to be subject to restrictive situational management strategies, it is reasonable to assume that the latter are often used in the absence of the former. This is clearly in conflict with the best practice principles outlined below.

Good practice in situational management

If situational management has to be employed, what principles should govern its use? Although emphases vary, a number of good practice points appear common across published international guidelines (Child Welfare League of America, 2004; Department of Health & Department for Education and Skills, 2002; Department of Human Services, 2009; Harris *et al.*, 2008; Welsh Assembly Government, 2005). These include the following.

- Situational management should only take place within a broader context of positive behavioural strategies designed to support people develop more appropriate adaptive behaviours and which focus on the prevention of challenging behaviour.
- There must be clear policies governing its general use in services and specific use with at-risk individuals.
- The application of situational management procedures must be clearly shown to be in the best interests of the service user concerned.
- Planned intervention is safer than unplanned and so, where known risks exist, the most appropriate responses should be agreed and incorporated into support plans on a pro-active basis.
- Whenever unplanned, emergency interventions have to be employed, their use should be subject to immediate review.
- Situational management should always involve the least-restrictive option, and with non-physical strategies always being used in preference to physical ones.
- Situational management strategies should not inadvertently reinforce challenging behaviour (for example, by the unintended delivery of contingent social attention).
- Carers should receive accredited training in situational management and this should be subject to regular updating.
- Physical strategies must employ the minimum force necessary to achieve safe control.

- They should not be aversive in nature (and specifically not involve the deliberate infliction of pain, the hyperextension of joints, or pressure on the neck, chest or back).
- Known high risk strategies (e.g. prone restraint) should not be employed.
- Physical management strategies should be employed for the minimum possible time.
- They should be subject to prior risk assessment, both from the perspective of the risks posed by the techniques *per se* and specific risks regarding their use with individuals with known pre-existing health problems
- They must be subject to regular internal and external review.
- They must always be followed by appropriate debriefing and post-incident support for both service users and carers

There is some limited evidence that policy guidance that stresses good practice principles of this nature can have a positive impact on care services (Murphy *et al.*, 2002).

The social validity of situational management strategies

The need to demonstrate social validity of interventions that was outlined in Chapter 2 applies as much to strategies designed to help manage challenging behaviours as it does to strategies designed to change such behaviours. It will be recalled that the three tests of social validity are that an intervention should (a) address a socially significant problem, (b) be undertaken in a manner which is acceptable to the main constituencies involved and (c) result in socially important outcomes or effects.

For the reasons already outlined in this chapter and elsewhere, there can be no doubt that challenging behaviours pose socially significant problems. Situational management strategies are therefore addressing problems with great social significance. But what of the other criteria?

Social acceptability?

There are very few studies that have sought to tap the views of people with intellectual disabilities in relation to the management of their challenging behaviour, and all were conducted in the UK. Murphy *et al.* sought the views of 26 people who had received treatment at a highly specialized hospital unit; 16 had experienced restraint and the same number seclusion (Murphy *et al.*, 1996). The majority of respondents reported negative reactions to both procedures. Sequeira and Halsted identified comparable results in interviews with five women who were placed in a secure psychiatric hospital (Sequeira and Halsted, 2001; Sequeira and Halstead, 2002). The interviews clearly captured the women's feelings about restraint (e.g. 'It really hurts', 'Is it *meant* to hurt, is it?', 'They put my hands behind my back. They were really pushing it, really angry about it') and about seclusion (e.g. 'It's cold in there. They've got no heating in there at all', 'I reckon some of the staff here might seclude people just to prove that they are in charge.'). Hawkins *et al.* reported similarly negative experiences from a community-based sample (e.g. 'Hurts ... legs, knees ... hurts knees, Sore', 'It hurts ... on my legs and on my ankles', 'They just put me down really ... too hard. I can't move. Just put me down gently.') (Hawkins *et al.*, 2005). Although the quotations from these last two studies are virtually interchangeable, the service in the Sequeira and Halstead paper utilized physical intervention techniques that were derived from the prison service model described above (and which therefore made use of pain-compliance procedures), whereas the service in the Hawkins *et al.* paper used an approach that rejected the use of such procedures and which aimed to be non-aversive in nature. This suggests that either physical interventions will be experienced as unpleasant by recipients irrespective of the intentions of their designers, or perhaps that even 'non-aversive' procedures may be implemented in an aggressive manner under the heat of field conditions. The one respondent in the latter study who had been subject to both approaches clearly viewed the new model as being less aversive, however, thus offering limited support for the development of less aversive methods. Jones and Kroese provided further evidence of the unacceptability of pain compliance procedures (e.g. 'Okay, but not bending your thumbs back. Didn't like that. It hurt.') (Jones and Kroese, 2006).

Three studies have directly attempted to measure the social validity of different types of physical intervention. McDonnell *et al.* found that university students, educational and residential care staff rated seated restraint as significantly more acceptable than two forms of floor restraint (McDonnell *et al.*, 1993; McDonnell and Sturmey, 2000). Cunningham *et al.* found that all three forms of restraint were rated negatively by groups of undergraduate students, care staff and people with intellectual disability, but that chair restraint was rated as the least aversive (Cunningham *et al.*, 2003). People with intellectual disabilities rated restraint more negatively than the other participant groups.

A small number have explored carer attitudes to the actual use of physical intervention with people who have intellectual disability. Staff interviewed by Hawkins *et al.* reported varying degrees of anticipatory anxiety as levels of individual's challenging behaviour escalated, positive (e.g. 'You're asserting control and preventing danger or preventing harm.') and negative feelings (e.g. 'It's very wearing ... the tension is physically exhausting', 'My level of stress rises as the service user struggles more and more.') during episodes of restraint and primarily negative feelings post-restraint (e.g. 'You're still on edge in case something happens again', 'Yesterday I was physically and emotionally drained after the intervention.') (Hawkins *et al.*, 2005). Staff interviewed by Edwards similarly reflected the stresses inherent in implementing restraint, but also the potential benefits of training (Edwards, 1999a, 1999b).

Socially significant outcomes?

Based on the discussion so far, a number of socially significant outcomes might be expected by including situational management strategies within behavioural support plans. These include: reduced rates of injury for both people with challenging behaviour and their carers, improved confidence in working with individuals who challenge, and improved competence in managing risk behaviours.

Unfortunately, both the quantity and quality of research into situational management strategies is extremely poor (and in the case of non-physical intervention strategies, virtually non-existent). This research has however been reviewed by a number of authors in recent years (Allen, 2001; McDonnell, 2009; Richter et al., 2006; Zarola and Leather, 2006), and it is possible to identify some emerging trends.

- Studies into different approaches to training carers in physical intervention that employ different designs and across different user groups provide reasonably consistent evidence that improved carer knowledge and confidence often result.
- In general, research tends to focus on the short-term, immediate consequences of training (e.g. trainee pre- and post-views) rather than more important, indirect (e.g. rates of injury) and long-term impacts.
- While some studies do suggest that training can impact positively on rates of challenging behaviour, rates of injuries, and workdays lost, overall, the data here are much less convincing.
- Training is likely to have most impact if it is delivered within broader organizational initiatives designed to reduce challenging behaviours.
- User views on socially valid outcomes are particularly lacking. While Jones and Kroese found that half of the respondents interviewed were able to recognize that physical intervention played a role in helping to prevent further risk to themselves or others (e.g. 'stops hurting yourself or others', 'stops you punching walls and hurting yourself') (Jones and Kroese, 2006), only a minority of users in Hawkins et al. expressed similar views (Hawkins et al., 2005).
- Research has focused almost exclusively on the outcomes of training paid carers, to the exclusion of family members.

While the difficulty of researching such a complex phenomenon is sometimes put forward as a defence for the paucity of empirical evidence in this area (Gaskin et al., 2007), this is ultimately an indefensible position given the known high-rate use of intrusive techniques that have the potential to pose significant risk (McDonnell, 2009; Sailas and Fenton, 1999). Bergk et al. have recently proposed a number of possible methodological templates for constructing randomized controlled trials of restraint and seclusion use (Bergk et al., 2008).

Reducing the use of situational management

While there is a clear place for situational management in behavioural intervention, the available research suggests that the use of restraint and seclusion with people who have intellectual disabilities and challenging behaviour is alarmingly and inappropriately high. Encouragingly, there is now a relatively substantial literature that both advocates for, and demonstrates the effectiveness of, organizational initiatives designed to reduce or eliminate the use of situational management strategies across a variety of vulnerable populations (Colton, 2008; Crosland et al., 2008; Miller et al., 2006; Paterson et al., 2008; Thompson et al., 2008). Several studies have been able to evidence substantial gains in terms of reduced staff and user injuries, sick leave, turnover and service costs.

There are several perspectives on how such outcomes can be achieved. At the most simple level, there is evidence that simply improved monitoring can significantly impact upon the rates of use of such procedures. For example, Rangecroft et al. reported a 29% reduction in restraint use in specialist treatment units and a 5% reduction in less-specialized residential units on a large hospital campus simply as a result of making staff aware that the use of such procedures was being monitored and scrutinized (Rangecroft et al., 1997). Second, there is evidence that the implementation of the behaviour change strategies described within this book can serve to reduce restraint use (Luiselli, 2009) as can interventions designed to improve psychological functioning in staff (Singh et al., 2006a; Singh et al., 2009b). Finally, there is evidence that more substantial multi-component organizational change strategies can also produce significant reductions and collateral positive benefits (Allen et al., 2003; Sanders, 2009; Sturmey and McGlyn, 2002). Suggested key organizational interventions include (Bullard et al., 2003; Huckshorn, 2005; Singh et al., 2006a; Singh et al., 2009b):

- leadership that prioritizes situational management reduction as a priority;
- the active involvement of supervisors and managers in reduction initiatives (e.g. by regularly reinforcing the organizational objective, modelling and coaching alternative approaches, etc.);
- the construction of clear organizational policies on situational management and the implementation of individualized behavioural support plans;
- proscribing the use of particular high-risk physical interventions;
- using data to monitor baseline practice and the impact of situational management initiatives;
- developing the workforce using competency-based approaches in critical areas such as prevention, de-escalation and appropriate, ethical situational management techniques;

- implementing effective debriefing procedures that are both supportive and ensuring that organizational learning follows both well-managed and less well-managed incidents of challenging behaviour;
- utilizing proactive approaches to manage staff stresses arising from working with challenging individuals;
- enhancing the role of service users in reduction interventions (e.g. by collecting feedback on the use of physical strategies as modelled in the research described above and by formally including them in committees, working groups, etc.);
- adopting formal quality assurance processes.

While all these suggestions appear intuitively correct and have good face validity, further research is necessary to identify those which are more critical in determining the outcomes described.

Summary

There are important clinical and ethical reasons for including guidelines for effective situational management within behavioural support plans. Despite a significant increase in the level of interest in this topic in recent years, it remains significantly under-researched and it is therefore not possible to draw firm conclusions about its social validity at the present time. There are at least three critical areas of work that remain to be addressed: much more widespread implementation of behaviour change strategies is required in order to reduce the need for situational management; more research is required on the development of ethically sound situational management techniques that are effective in managing challenging behaviour and which enhance the safety of both the individual with challenging behaviour and their carers; and, a greater understanding of, and commitment to, providing service cultures that insulate against inappropriate use of such techniques is urgently needed.

Challenges ahead: adopting an evidence-based public health approach to challenging behaviour

The last four decades has witnessed dramatic advances in our understanding of challenging behaviours shown by people with severe intellectual disabilities. We have learned that many (but certainly not all) challenging behaviours are, at least in the short term, functional and adaptive responses to challenging contexts. We have begun to understand something of the complexity that underlies the emergence and persistence of challenging behaviours. We have begun to develop a range of interventions with demonstrable efficacy and, in some countries, establish systems for the delivery of these interventions to people with intellectual disabilities who show challenging behaviours. There remain, however, some significant challenges ahead.

Perhaps the greatest of these challenges is to develop an evidence-based public health approach to challenging behaviours. Public health has been defined as 'the science and art of preventing disease, prolonging life and promoting health through the organized efforts and informed choices of society, organizations, public and private, communities and individuals' (Winslow, 1920). In our context it would involve the implementation of a co-ordinated set of health and social policies to reduce the incidence and prevalence of challenging behaviours among people with severe intellectual disabilities. Such an approach moves far beyond the issue of scaling up the delivery of efficacious interventions to fully embrace the notion of prevention. But such an approach needs to be evidence based, and that in itself represents a significant challenge to this research community. In the following section we briefly review the types of evidence that are necessary to inform the development of such an approach. We then discuss some potential components of a public-health or population-level approach to challenging behaviours.

Evidence of what?

Archie Cochrane identified three types or levels of evidence that are required to inform health policy: efficacy, effectiveness and efficiency (Cochrane, 1972).

Challenging Behaviour, 3rd edn, ed. Eric Emerson and Stewart L. Einfeld. Published by Cambridge University Press. © E. Emerson and S. L. Einfeld 2011.

Efficacy is the extent to which an intervention achieves its intended aims under ideal or near ideal circumstances. Effectiveness (or impact, see below) assesses whether an intervention actually achieves its intended aims when provided under the typical conditions of practice in a given country at a given point in time. Efficiency measures the effect of an intervention in relation to the resources involved through, for example, cost effectiveness or cost benefit studies. Evidence of efficiency is the most relevant type of information when faced with decisions about investing in alternative policies, service configurations or interventions. Put more colloquially the three levels can be translated into three key questions (Haynes, 1999):

- Can it work?
- Does it work?
- Is it worth it?

When these frameworks are applied to knowledge regarding approaches to supporting people with intellectual disabilities and challenging behaviours, the inescapable conclusion must be that we have amassed an impressive body of evidence on the short-term *efficacy* of behavioural interventions. It has been demonstrated beyond doubt, for example, that positive behaviour support can bring about short- to medium-term reductions in challenging behaviours. Beyond that, however, evidence in this field is sparse indeed (Emerson, 2006). The *ad hoc* accumulation of case studies (however sophisticated the methodology) by high-profile well-resourced research and development centres tells us nothing about either effectiveness or efficiency. Evidence of efficacy only tells us about impact, and often only under very advantageous circumstances. A highly efficacious intervention may be ineffective and inefficient if uptake or compliance is low or the duration of benefits short.

There are, of course, some significant practical difficulties associated with testing the effectiveness and efficiency of interventions. This is, however, the type of information most valuable when attempting to shape health and social policy. The difficulties are not, however, insurmountable. One very pragmatic way forward is the generation of 'practice-based evidence' through the systematic generation of evidence from routine practice (Barkham and Mellor-Clark, 2003; Bergstrom, 2008; Green, 2006; McDonald and Viehbeck, 2007). In this era of 'evidence-based practice' and public service accountability, the systematic monitoring of the actual outcomes delivered by services is increasingly considered to be a fundamental requisite of 'good practice'. The co-ordination of information generated through such activity can go some way to building a much needed body of evidence on effectiveness. This is a critically important issue for the field, as the absence of evidence on effectiveness and efficiency is a significant barrier to securing the level of investment necessary to scale up the delivery of effective supports to people with intellectual disabilities and their families who need it.

Within a public health framework, evidence of impact would be based on the extent to which the delivery of scaled-up interventions changed the population-level prevalence of challenging behaviours among people with intellectual disability. Impact is a measure of effectiveness when applied to public health programmes that seek to change population (rather than individual) health. In 1996 Abrams and Orleans *et al.* defined the impact of an intervention as the product of the percentage of the population receiving it (reach) and its effectiveness (impact = R X E) (Abrams *et al.*, 1996). Glasgow and colleagues subsequently expanded this definition to include three further dimensions in order to fully characterize a population level of impact: adoption, implementation and maintenance (Glasgow *et al.*, 1999). These five dimensions (RE-AIM) provide a framework in which to evaluate community-based public health interventions. Each dimension can be represented on a 0%–100% scale and the impact is derived from the combined effects of the five dimensions. *Adoption* is similar to reach, but is evaluated at the level of the settings that are potentially involved in delivery of services to the target population. *Implementation* refers to the capacity to ensure that the program is delivered as it is intended. *Maintenance* is concerned with the longer-term effects of the program on targeted outcomes, both for the agency that delivers the program and the people, families or communities that participate.

A public-health approach to challenging behaviour

Key components of a public health approach to challenging behaviours can be considered within frameworks of prevention (Allen *et al.*, in press). Traditionally, it has been common practice to distinguish three levels of prevention (Caplan, 1964; World Health Organization, 2004).

- *Primary prevention* strategies would seek to eliminate or reduce the prevalence of challenging behaviours by reducing the probability of it initially occurring. In a similar manner, the provisions of adequate sanitation and housing conditions are primary preventative strategies for the reduction of health conditions associated with a range of infectious diseases.
- *Secondary prevention* strategies would seek to eliminate or reduce the prevalence of challenging behaviours by intervening in the early stages of their development. The widespread investment in primary health care is an example of a policy based on general ideas of secondary prevention.
- *Tertiary prevention* strategies would seek to eliminate or reduce challenging behaviours by providing effective support to people who already show challenging behaviours. Tertiary prevention is the realm of clinical intervention and support services.

While this framework has been criticized on the mismatch of the three distinct phases suggested and the rather messier reality of the developmental trajectories of emotional and behavioural difficulties (Vitaro and Tremblay, 2008), it still provides a useful heuristic in the present context for identifying preventative options. Prevention science (Coie *et al.*, 2000), which is primarily concerned with primary and secondary prevention in the above framework, typically distinguishes between programmes on the basis of who is offered the intervention (Offord and Bennett, 2002; Vitaro and Tremblay, 2008).

- *Universal strategies* are delivered to whole populations (e.g. the mandatory use of safety belts, fluoridization of the water supply). The term quasi-universal is sometimes used to describe programmes delivered to all individuals within a geographical area or institution (e.g. school) (Groark and McCall, 2008).
- *Targeted strategies* are delivered to specific sub-groups who are considered particularly at risk for the development of the condition or problem. These can be further subdivided into *selective* and *indicated*. *Selective strategies* are delivered to population sub-groups identified on the basis of their increased environmental risk of adverse outcomes (e.g. *Sure Start* programmes that are targeted at families living in materially and socially deprived areas). *Indicated strategies* are delivered to individuals identified on the basis of individual characteristics associated with increased risk of adverse outcomes (e.g. parenting classes for families supporting children with early signs of conduct difficulties).

Given the overlap between primary and secondary prevention, we will address both areas together prior to discussing tertiary prevention.

Primary and secondary prevention

Seccombe differentiates between preventative initiatives designed to 'change the odds' and those designed to 'beat the odds' of a condition developing (Seccombe, 2002). The former are interventions that are designed to reduce levels of exposure to known risk factors for the development of a problem. The latter are designed to foster the development of protective capacity and resilience (or reduce vulnerability) when exposed to known risk factors. In terms of the model described above, while primary prevention is essentially concerned with both 'changing the odds' (by reducing exposure to risk) and 'beating the odds' (by building generalized resilience), secondary and tertiary prevention focus solely on 'beating the odds'.

Changing the odds: universal strategies

Our growing knowledge of the determinants of challenging behaviours suggests a number of universal primary preventative strategies have the potential to reduce the prevalence of challenging behaviours among people with intellectual disability. Below we give two general examples.

First, exposure to adversity (e.g. socio-economic, stressful life events, abuse) is associated with significantly higher rates of emotional and behavioural difficulties among people with intellectual disability (Emerson and Einfeld, 2010; Emerson and Hatton, 2007d; Emerson *et al.*, 2010; Hulbert-Williams and Hastings, 2008). Evidence from the study of behavioural difficulties among children in general suggests that exposure to adversity has a causal influence on the emergence and persistence of behavioural difficulties (Glaser, 2008; Jenkins, 2008; Jones, 2008; Sandberg and Rutter, 2008; Tremblay, 2000; Tremblay *et al.*, 2004; Tremblay, 2006). As such, social policies that significantly reduce levels of exposure to adversity should have an impact on reducing the prevalence of challenging behaviours. Potential examples would include social policies that effectively reduce child poverty rates or reduce levels of violence within communities and families (Prinz *et al.*, 2009). At present, no studies have attempted to measure the impact of such initiatives on the prevalence of challenging behaviours among people with intellectual disability. There is, however, evidence from quasi-experimental studies that reductions in poverty within communities is associated with reduced rates of child emotional and behavioural difficulties (Costello *et al.*, 2003).

Second, we have seen above that some instances of challenging behaviours shown by people with severe intellectual disability can be conceptualized as adaptive communicative responses. As such, universal strategies that enhance the communicative capacity of children with severe intellectual disabilities should have an impact on reducing the prevalence of challenging behaviours. Potential examples would include the provision of pre-school education or in-home support that effectively enhanced the communicative abilities of all children with severe intellectual disabilities. Again, however, we are not aware of any studies that have attempted to measure the impact of such initiatives on the prevalence of challenging behaviours among people with intellectual disability.

Changing the odds: targeted strategies
Either of the above strategies could also constitute potentially effective targeted strategies to prevention if applied to high-risk populations (e.g. families supporting a child with intellectual disability living in poverty, children with early signs of challenging behaviours). In addition, the last two decades has seen significant investment in the development of targeted parent support programmes to reduce behavioural difficulties shown by children in general. These include both *selective strategies* (delivered to population sub-groups identified on the basis of their increased environmental risk, e.g. families living in poverty) or *indicated strategies* (delivered to the families of children showing early signs of conduct difficulties). The available evidence suggests that such interventions can be highly effective in reducing the prevalence of conduct difficulties (Boisjoli *et al.*, 2007; Burger, 2010; Churchill and Clarke, 2009; de Graaf *et al.*, 2008a, 2008b; Dishion *et al.*, 2008; Doyle *et al.*, 2009; Durlak and Wells, 1998; Hosman *et al.*, 2005; Irwin *et al.*, 2007; Mercy and Saul, 2009;

Mihalopoulos *et al.*, 2007; Offord and Bennett, 2002; Petitclerc and Tremblay, 2009; Prinz *et al.*, 2009; Ramey and Ramey, 1998; Reynolds *et al.*, 2007; Sanders, 2008; Thomas and Zimmer-Gembeck, 2007; Tremblay, 2006; Turner and Sanders, 2006; US Department of Health and Human Services, 2010; Vitaro and Tremblay, 2008; Webster-Stratton and Taylor, 2001; Webster-Stratton *et al.*, 2008; Zubrick *et al.*, 2005). There is also growing evidence that such approaches may prove effective in improving the emotional and behavioural well-being of children with (or at risk of) intellectual disability (Chasson *et al.*, 2007; Eldevik *et al.*, 2009; Guralnick, 1997, 2005; Harris *et al.*, 1991; McConachie and Diggle, 2007; McIntyre, 2008a, 2008b; Ramey and Ramey, 1998; Remington *et al.*, 2007).

For example, Stepping Stones Triple P (SSTP) is a public health strategy to reduce the prevalence of behavioural difficulties among children with intellectual or developmental disability (Sanders *et al.*, 2004). Based on the Triple P system, it involves five levels of intervention on a tiered continuum of increasing strength and narrowing population reach.

- Level 1 involves a universal parent and professional information media strategies with web-based materials to increase the receptivity of parents of a child with intellectual or developmental disability to participating in the programme (Sanders and Turner, 2002).
- Level 2 involves three 90-minute sessions with standardized presentations and self-directed use of programme materials delivered in a large group format (e.g. primary school).
- Level 3 (Primary Care Stepping Stones) involves a four-session intervention with a primary health-care provider (e.g. child health nurse, GP, school counsellor) including active skills training for a discrete child problem.
- Level 4 involves an intensive 8- to 10-session individual or group parent-training programme combining information with active skills training across a broad range of target behaviours in both home and community settings.
- Level 5 involves an enhanced parent-training programme for families experiencing both parenting problems and other sources of stress. This is an optional addition to the standard programme for those parents who continue to experience difficulty in implementing strategies.

The Triple P system meets the standards-of-evidence criteria for dissemination outlined by the Society for Prevention Research (Society for Prevention Research., 2004): there is a substantial body of evidence of efficacy and effectiveness; the system has the capacity to go to scale with professionally developed resource materials and a standardized training and accreditation process for service providers; there is clear and readily available information relating to cost-effectiveness; evaluation tools are available; and conditions necessary to sustain the programme and assure quality is maintained have been identified (de Graaf *et al.*, 2008a, 2008b; Mercy and Saul, 2009; Mihalopoulos *et al.*, 2007;

Prinz *et al.*, 2009; Sanders, 2008; Thomas and Zimmer-Gembeck, 2007; Turner and Sanders, 2006; Zubrick *et al.*, 2005).

While Stepping Stones Triple P (SSTP) has not yet been subject to as many studies as its Triple P parent, there have been three randomized controlled trials (RCT) of efficacy. Roberts and colleagues, in an RCT with 47 families with children with intellectual disability, reported that SSTP was associated with reductions in child behaviour problems both by parent report and observational data (Roberts *et al.*, 2006). Plant and Saunders, in an RCT involving the parents of 74 pre-school aged children with developmental disabilities, reported that SSTP was associated with lower levels of observed child behaviour problems, and improved parent report of competence and satisfaction in the parenting role compared with a wait-list condition. The reductions in child behaviour difficulties were significant and clinically reliable for 67% of children and were maintained at 1-year follow-up (Plant and Sanders, 2007). Finally, a third RCT involving the parents of 59 children with autism spectrum disorders, reported a reduction in parent-reported child behaviour problems and dysfunctional parenting styles (Whittingham *et al.*, 2009). One-third of the children showed clinically reliable change on the measures of child problem behaviour and changes were maintained at 6-month follow-up.

This evidence, from studies involving children with and without intellectual disability, suggests that scaling up the delivery (reach) of targeted parent support/education programmes could have a significant impact on reducing the prevalence of behavioural difficulties and challenging behaviours among children with intellectual disability. There is a long history, however, of effective public health programmes, while increasing health overall, also widening inequalities in health within populations (White *et al.*, 2009). Indeed, there is evidence that targeted parent support/education programmes may be less effective for disadvantaged parents (Harris *et al.*, 1991; Lundahl *et al.*, 2006) and concern that they may serve to locate the causes of social exclusion in individual characteristics, rather than social processes (Churchill and Clarke, 2009). Ensuring that targeted preventative strategies do not increase inequity will primarily require ensuring that such services have equitable reach and maintenance. Vitaro and Tremblay identify key components of effective targeted interventions and key strategies to ensure widespread and equitable reach, adoption and maintenance (Vitaro and Tremblay, 2008).

Beating the odds: promoting resilience
While reducing exposure to risk factors associated with the emergence or persistence of challenging behaviours represents an optimal strategy, it is clear that exposure to all risks cannot be eliminated. As such, it becomes important to consider preventative interventions that aim to promote individual, family and community resilience in the face of adversity, or, in Seccombe's phrase to help people 'beat the odds' (Seccombe, 2002). There exists an

extensive literature on the biological, personal and contextual factors associated with childhood resilience in the face of adversity (Broberg *et al.*, 2009; Burchardt and Huerta, 2008; Coleman and Hagell, 2007; Friedli, 2009; Goldstein and Brooks, 2006; Jenkins, 2008; Luthar *et al.*, 2000; Luthar, 2003, 2006; Luthar *et al.*, 2006; Luthar and Brown, 2007; Rutter, 1979, 1985, 1987, 1999; Sandberg and Rutter, 2008; Schoon, 2006; Ungar, 2008). Potential resilience-enhancing interventions of perhaps particular relevance to people with intellectual disability include intervention in childhood and throughout the lifecourse that aim to promote:

- positive achievements
- self-esteem
- empowerment
- problem solving
- social skills relevant to friendship formation and maintenance
- inclusive social relationships through employment, volunteering and other forms of social participation.

Examples of strategies that may result in such outcomes include:

- having control over a personal budget, with appropriate support for planning
- participation in self-advocacy groups
- supported employment
- participation in artistic and sporting activities
- volunteering.

Unfortunately, whilst such supports/interventions are often advocated, remarkably little empirical research has been undertaken to evaluate their impact. However, a small number (of often methodologically questionable studies) suggest that participation in activities that may help build self-esteem or may give a sense of achievement (e.g. sporting activities, challenging outdoor adventure activities) may be associated with greater well-being (Carmeli *et al.*, 2008; Dykens and Cohen, 1996; Maiano *et al.*, 2001; Ninot *et al.*, 2005; Rose and Massey, 1993; Weiss and Bebko, 2008).

Tertiary prevention

Enhancing tertiary prevention services for people with intellectual disability and challenging behaviours will require the scaling up of systems to effectively deliver interventions, which evidence suggests can reduce the severity, halt the progression or minimize the impact of challenging behaviours once they are established. In previous chapters we have briefly reviewed the evidence of efficacy of a range of interventions. This, when combined with current know-ledge regarding the determinants of challenging behaviours, suggests that no single approach to intervention (e.g. medication, positive behaviour support) will be effective in all instances. As such, it is critical that intervention approaches need to be functionally based. That is, they need to be tailored to the specific factors that are predisposing, precipitating and maintaining the challenging behaviour of that particular individual in the contexts in which they live. At present, however, the weight of evidence does support the adoption of positive behaviour support as the approach of first choice (Ball *et al.*, 2004; Campbell, 2003; Didden *et al.*, 1997; Didden *et al.*, 2006; Harvey *et al.*, 2009; Marquis *et al.*, 2000; Scotti *et al.*, 1991b).

The need to scale up delivery of these 'promising practices' is clear. In all countries there exists an enormous gap between knowledge concerning effective approaches and the routine availability of such approaches in educational, health and social services (Department of Health, 1993, 2007). At present, the majority of people who show challenging behaviour do not receive effective behavioural support (Emerson *et al.*, 2000; Emerson, 2001b; Oliver *et al.*, 1987; Qureshi, 1994; Stancliffe *et al.*, 1999), even among people receiving residential supports from 'better' providers (Emerson *et al.*, 2000).

In the following section we discuss some of the factors that are likely to support or impede the scaling-up of tertiary prevention services. First, however, we will briefly discuss the often vexed question of the nature and location of tertiary support systems.

The location and organization of tertiary support systems
Much has been written over recent years about the viability and relative effectiveness of local community-based and centre or unit-based approaches to delivering and sustaining interventions and supports for people with severe challenging behaviours (Blunden and Allen, 1987; Department of Health, 1993, 2007). In large part, this discussion reflects the continuing legacy of our historical investment in large-scale segregated institutional residential provision for people with intellectual disabilities. While reliance on such services for residential support has markedly diminished in many countries, they have continued to serve a residual role in relation to the treatment and management of challenging behaviours and mental health problems in many instances. Two issues are important here. First, how can tertiary intervention services be best delivered? Second, how can the long-term residential support of people who show persistent serious challenging behaviours be best organized?

Delivering interventions
Following the logic of investment in primary health care, local community-based systems for delivering interventions must be considered the preferred option for the delivery of health care (World Health Organization, 2008a). Community-based primary care delivery systems minimize cost and inconvenience to service users and allow for assessment and intervention to take place in the natural settings within which people live, learn, work and play. The latter is particularly important in the present context, given that many challenging

behaviours appear to be intimately connected to everyday environmental conditions. A number of studies have investigated the effectiveness of different
approaches to providing short- to medium-term intervention services for
people with severe challenging behaviour (Allen and Felce, 1999). The evidence
from these suggests that, while peripatetic community-based intervention
services are capable of providing effective behavioural support through a
process of consultation to community-based services (and may be preferable
to centre or unit-based alternatives), their effectiveness may be less than
optimal in a substantial proportion of cases (Allen and Felce, 1999; Emerson
et al., 1996a; Hassiotis et al., 2009; Hudson et al., 1995; Lowe et al., 1996).
Failures in the reach and effectiveness of peripatetic community-based intervention services have contributed to the continuing social exclusion of people
with intellectual disabilities and challenging behaviours and created a market to
the development and maintenance of larger and less inclusive assessment and
treatment units (Department of Health, 1993, 2007; Emerson and Robertson,
2008). However, such provision is indicative of system failure (rather than
reflecting the 'need' of people with intellectual disability).

Long-term support
Over the last two decades, a range of (then) innovative projects have helped
demonstrate the viability and benefits of providing long-term support to people
with severe challenging behaviour in small more inclusive community-based
settings (Cameron et al., 1998; Emerson et al., 1994; Mansell et al., 2001; Risley,
1996). Two distinct (though complementary) rationales underlie the development of long-term community-based supports for people with severe challenging behaviour. First, it has been argued that people with severe challenging
behaviour have as legitimate an entitlement as all other people with intellectual
disabilities to a decent quality of life. From this basis, supports may be developed to maximize quality of life *regardless* of the extent of challenging behaviour shown by the individual. Second, developing community-based supports
may be considered a 'molar' approach to the antecedent control of challenging
behaviour (Carr et al., 1998). That is, it has been suggested that the provision of
high quality community-based supports should be seen as an integral component of effective intervention (Cameron et al., 1998; Risley, 1996). In addition, a
number of studies have specifically examined the outcomes associated with
small community-based residential supports for people with severe challenging
behaviour (Allen and Felce, 1999). These studies have demonstrated that: (1) it
is possible to establish and maintain such services, even for those people
considered to present the greatest challenge to services (Department of
Health, 1993, 2007; Emerson, 1990; Emerson et al., 1994; Mansell et al.,
2001); (2) the outcomes associated with such services are typically superior to
those associated with institutional provision (Department of Health, 1993,
2007; Felce et al., 1998; Golding et al., 2005; Knobbe et al., 1995; Mansell

et al., 2001). There also exists a substantial international literature that has consistently reported that, while deinstitutionalization is not necessarily associated with a decrease in challenging behaviour, people living in community-based residential supports, including people with challenging behaviour, experience a better overall quality of life than people supported in either institutional or medium-sized residential provision (Emerson and Hatton, 1994, 1996; Kim *et al.*, 2001; Kozma *et al.*, 2009; Walsh *et al.*, 2008; Young *et al.*, 1998). Taken together, these sources of evidence suggest that long-term support for people with severe intellectual disability and challenging behaviours who no longer live with their family should be provided in small inclusive community-based settings (Department of Health, 2007; Emerson and Robertson, 2008). Again, more remote or more institutional provision must be seen as indicative of system failure (rather than the 'need' of people with intellectual disability).

Scaling up services

Scaling up (or extending the reach of) services and interventions (whether preventative or tertiary) will require the development or expansion of effective delivery systems. In the following sections we will briefly address some key general issues involved in scaling up health services and the adoption of innovation. It is important to keep in mind, however, that the specific config-uration of services and supports will always need to be responsive to, and will reflect, local cultural, economic and policy contexts.

Simmons and Shiffman provide a thoughtful discussion of four key elements involved in successfully scaling up innovative health care interventions: (1) the innovation itself; (2) the 'resource team' of individuals or institutions advocating its wider use; (3) the potential adopting organization(s); and (4) the strategies employed for scaling-up (Simmons and Shiffman, 2007). They also identify key attributes for each of these elements that are likely to facilitate successful scaling-up.

The innovation

Glaser and others have identified key characteristics of innovations that appear to facilitate their transfer to practice (Glaser *et al.*, 1983). They suggested that adoption will be facilitated if innovations:

- are based on sound evidence (or are promoted by credible people or institutions);
- deliver observable results;
- are relevant for addressing important problems;
- have a relative advantage over existing practices;
- are easy to adopt, implement and understand;

- are compatible with the potential users' established values, norms and facilities;
- can be tested out by potential adopting organizations prior to committing to complete adoption.

When judged against such criteria, it is clear that positive behaviour support faces some significant barriers to adoption. As we have seen above:

- evidence of effectiveness or efficiency is lacking and, as such, the advantage over existing practices is difficult to establish;
- positive behaviour support is not easy to adopt or implement as a tertiary intervention, though its growing systemic use in mainstream school systems suggests it can provide a viable approach to prevention (Horner *et al.*, 2009); and
- the social validity or acceptability of behavioural interventions is questionable in many settings.

To facilitate adoption, it will be important to address the first and last of these three issues by generating evidence of effectiveness and efficiency that is credible to major stakeholders and continuing to work to promote acceptability, values and 'humane face' of positive behaviour support (Carr, 2007). Critically important is that actual practices maximize the 'goodness of fit' with key aspects of the context in which they are to be implemented (Albin *et al.*, 1996; Lucyshyn *et al.*, 2002; Singer *et al.*, 2002) and are socio-culturally relevant and engaging (Chen *et al.*, 2002; Hatton *et al.*, 2010; Netto *et al.*, 2010; Vitaro and Tremblay, 2008). Netto and colleagues have identified five principles for adapting behavioural interventions for minority ethnic communities (Netto *et al.*, 2010):

1. use community resources to publicize the intervention and increase accessibility;
2. identify and address barriers to access and participation;
3. develop communication strategies which are sensitive to language use and information requirements;
4. work with cultural or religious values that either promote or hinder behavioural change; and
5. accommodate varying degrees of cultural identification.

It has also been suggested that this will be more likely if a behavioural 'support plan and its components are consistent with or highly compatible with the values and skills of key stakeholders and plan implementors; readily sustainable given the resources and constraints of the environments, conditions and systems where the plan is implemented; and suitable to the unique needs of the person with problem behaviors' (Albin *et al.*, 1996, pp. 82–83). In practice, the idea of 'contextual fit' (which has clear links to ideas of social validity and feasibility analysis) means that ideally:

- the goals of intervention should be developed in partnership with the person with intellectual disabilities and those supporting them;
- the form of intervention should reflect the culture, values and the skills available or potentially available to the people who will be implementing the intervention plan;

- the detailed activities required for programme implementation should enmesh with existing routines and activity patterns;
- the requirements of appropriate implementation are feasible within the constraints and competing demands operating on the people who will be responsible for implementation.

The 'resource team'

Simmons and Shiffman use the term 'resource team' to refer to those individuals or institutions involved in the development of an innovation who are also active in advocating its wider use (Simmons and Shiffman, 2007). They suggest that resource teams involved in the promotion of the innovation are more likely to be successful if they:
- include effective and motivated leaders who command authority and have credibility with potential adopting organizations;
- have a unifying vision;
- appreciate the capacities and limitations of potential adopting organizations;
- understand the political, social and cultural environments within which scaling up is to take place;
- have the ability to generate resources; and
- have the relevant technical skills, training capacity and management skills.

Unfortunately, it is difficult in many, if not most, countries to identify a 'resource team' that comes close to meeting these criteria.

The adopting organization(s)

Simmons and Shiffman suggest that successful transfer of innovations is facilitated when potential adopting organizations have the following characteristics (Simmons and Shiffman, 2007):
- key leaders in potential adopting organizations perceive the innovation to represent a timely and viable solution to a current or pending significant problem;
- the organization has effective leadership and the requisite implementation capacity;
- the resource team and potential adopting organizations share similar characteristics and are in reasonably close physical proximity.

The scaling-up strategy

Finally, Simmons and Shiffman suggest that successful transfer of innovation to practice is more likely to occur when the scaling-up strategy has the following characteristics (Simmons and Shiffman, 2007):
- the advantages of adopting the innovation are made clearly visible to key stakeholders through a process of participatory action-orientated evaluation process;

- there is frequent and positive personal contact and informal communication between the resource team and the adopting organization;
- members of the adopting organization are involved early on in the development of a scaling-up strategy;
- the innovation is adapted to the local context and introduced on a time-scale sensitive to available resources;
- the adopting organization receives supportive technical assistance;
- there is an ongoing focus on sustainability.

Evidence suggests that many approaches to intervention may either need to be sustained over considerable periods of time or require permanent changes in patterns of interaction between people with intellectual disabilities and those who support them. This does not mean that significant reductions in challenging behaviour are not possible over the short term. On the contrary, most of the approaches to providing effective behavioural support have been shown, under certain circumstances, to bring about rapid and socially valid improvements in the situations of people who show severe challenging behaviour. However, maintaining these gains, generalizing them to new settings and achieving broader 'lifestyle' outcomes are unlikely to occur without sustained support. Indeed, some approaches (e.g. the functional displacement of challenging behaviour through supporting the use of more appropriate communicative acts) requires permanent changes in the behaviour of carers and support staff. As has been pointed out, 'patterns of severe challenging behaviours do not simply 'disappear'. Long-term support plans must create and maintain settings and programmatic contexts in which these behaviors are made and continue to be ineffective, inefficient, or irrelevant. Only then will near-zero levels of challenging behaviors occur and be maintained in all settings relevant to a person's life' (Anderson *et al.*, 1993).

Such a requirement does, of course, pose a major challenge to the organization of support systems. This should not, however, surprise us. The behavioural approach suggests that challenging behaviours have been shaped over time, and are currently being maintained by powerful contingencies of reinforcement. We should expect that, unless intervention brings about a *lasting change* in the maintaining contingencies, intervention gains are unlikely to prove durable. As we have seen, establishing alternative behaviours is only likely to be effective if the person's challenging behaviour is made 'ineffective, inefficient, or irrelevant'. Intervention needs to be seen as an ongoing process, rather than as a time-limited episode of 'treatment'.

This perspective forces us to consider ways in which intervention can bring about sustained changes in the ways in which carers and care staff interact with people with learning disabilities. It requires us to address the various sources of influences operating on carers and care staff including: the resources available to families or in community settings; competing demands on the time and energy of carers and care staff; the beliefs and attitudes they hold about the person's challenging behaviours; and the ways in which these beliefs are shaped, supported and translated into action. Given that carers are themselves likely to experience strong emotional reactions and heightened stress levels (Bromley and Emerson, 1995; Cottle *et al.*, 1995), it will also be important to provide effective emotional and practical support to front-line carers. Promising initial research suggests that the addition of mindfulness-based interventions with paid carers can enhance the impact of behavioural training and produce improved outcomes in terms of reduced rates of challenging behaviour, restraint and emergency medication use, and staff and service user injuries (Noone and Hastings, in press; Singh *et al.*, 2006a; Singh *et al.*, 2006b; Singh *et al.*, 2009b).

The balance of investment

We believe there are strong arguments in support of adopting a more preventative population-level 'public health' approach to challenging behaviours. There is also growing evidence from elsewhere that such an approach is both viable and effective in reducing behavioural problems shown by children in general (Boisjoli *et al.*, 2007; Burger, 2010; Churchill and Clarke, 2009; de Graaf *et al.*, 2008a, 2008b; Dishion *et al.*, 2008; Doyle *et al.*, 2009; Durlak and Wells, 1998; Hosman *et al.*, 2005; Irwin *et al.*, 2007; Mercy and Saul, 2009; Mihalopoulos *et al.*, 2007; Offord and Bennett, 2002; Petitclerc and Tremblay, 2009; Prinz *et al.*, 2009; Ramey and Ramey, 1998; Reynolds *et al.*, 2007; Sanders, 2008; Thomas and Zimmer-Gembeck, 2007; Tremblay, 2006; Turner and Sanders, 2006; Vitaro and Tremblay, 2008; Webster-Stratton and Taylor, 2001; Webster-Stratton *et al.*, 2008; Zubrick *et al.*, 2005). There are also, of course, strong arguments in support of scaling up the delivery of effective support and interventions to people with serious and persistent challenging behaviours and growing evidence of the efficacy of certain approaches area (Ball *et al.*, 2004; Campbell, 2003; Didden *et al.*, 1997; Didden *et al.*, 2006; Harvey *et al.*, 2009; Lang *et al.*, 2009b; Marquis *et al.*, 2000; Scotti *et al.*, 1991b).

The reality, however, is that resources for the support of people with intellectual disabilities will always be rationed, and at times significantly so. As a result, difficult choices need to be made regarding the relative benefits of alternative approaches. As we have pointed out on several occasions, the current lack of evidence on the effectiveness and efficiency of alternative approaches makes taking such decisions problematic. One consequence of these problems regarding the evidence-base of interventions is that health and social care services tend to opt for default positions; primarily investing resources in a largely unplanned (and potentially ineffective) manner in response to individual crises. While the generation of better evidence may not prevent the inefficient use of scarce resources, it could make a positive contribution to moving towards a more rational and effective approach to supporting people with intellectual disabilities and challenging behaviours.

Some final thoughts

Broadening perspectives

Updating this book after a decade has been an interesting, and at times frustrating, experience. Both previous editions, in their concluding sections, stressed the importance of developing more integrated and broader approaches to understanding challenging behaviours (Emerson, 1995, 2001a). Those words appear just as relevant today as they were 10 and 15 years ago. All too often we continue to work within our conceptual silos.

That is not to say that no progress has been made. It has. There are now some excellent examples of the integration of biological and behavioural approaches to understanding challenging behaviours (Horsler and Oliver, 2006); positive behaviour support has emerged and expanded to embrace links with hedonic psychology and notions of quality of life (Carr, 2007); we have learned much more about the natural trajectories of challenging behaviours over time (Einfeld *et al.*, 2006); and we have begun to attend to the potentially important role of social context on the prevalence and persistence of challenging behaviours (Emerson and Hatton, 2007d; Emerson and Einfeld, 2010).

It is still very evident, however, that there exist some marked discrepancies between the models, theories and approaches applied to understanding behavioural difficulties shown by people with and without intellectual disability. Why in our attempt to understand challenging behaviours shown by children with intellectual disability do family dynamics, relationships and attachments appear so invisible? Why do we pay so little attention to the role that neighbourhoods and communities play in the emergence and persistent of challenging behaviours? While the situation of children with intellectual disability is different from other children, are they so 'other' that ideas and knowledge about what helps determine the well-being of 'typically developing' children are irrelevant to our interests? That is, of course, a rhetorical question. Perhaps it is time for the research and practice communities focusing on challenging behaviours shown by people with intellectual disabilities to look up and take note of broader developments in our understanding of troublesome behaviour (Rutter *et al.*, 2008; Tremblay, 2000).

Challenging behaviours in low and middle income countries

Last, but far from least, it is notable that *all* of the evidence cited in this book has been generated within the world's richer countries (and primarily within the world's richer English-speaking countries). Yet, of the 6.69 billion people in the world today, just 16% live in high-income economies, and only 6% live in high-income Anglophone economies (World Bank, 2010). Given that there are good reasons to believe that the incidence, and possibly prevalence, of intellectual disability will be higher in poorer nations (Durkin, 2002; Emerson *et al.*, 2007a; Institute of Medicine, 2001), it is reasonable to assume that the majority of people with severe intellectual disability and challenging behaviours also live in the world's low and middle income countries, countries in which health care resources are in desperately short supply (Patel *et al.*, 2007a; Patel *et al.*, 2007b; Saraceno *et al.*, 2007; World Health Organization, 2008b).

Of course, much of the evidence cited in this book that addresses basic biological or psychological processes is likely to transcend national and cultural boundaries. However, evidence relating to the relative influence of the broader determinants of challenging behaviours is unlikely to have cross-cultural validity, and issues relating to service development and delivery will certainly have to reflect the economic, cultural and social context of the countries in which they are to be delivered. Key issues in scaling up service delivery in low and middle income countries include the development of low-cost and culturally sensitive procedures for identifying people with intellectual disabilities, and extending the reach and effectiveness of community-based rehabilitation and family-centred support to people with intellectual disabilities and the families who support them (Einfeld *et al.*, 2009; Emerson *et al.*, 2008; Robertson *et al.*, 2009a; Robertson *et al.*, 2009b; World Health Organization, 2008b). The inclusion of intellectual disability in the World Health Organization's Mental Health Gap Action Programme aims to address these issues and will, hopefully, provide opportunities for the international research and practice communities to adopt a more global perspective in their work (World Health Organization, 2008b).

References

Aber, J. L., Bennett, N. G., Conley, D. C. and Li, J. (1997). The effects of poverty on child health and development. *Annual Review of Public Health*, **18**, 463–483.

Abrams, D. B., Orleans, C. T., Niaura, R. S., Goldstein, M. G., Prochaska, J. O. and Velicer, W. (1996). Integrating individual and public health perspectives for treatment of tobacco dependence under managed health care: a combined stepped-care and matching model. *Annals of Behavioral Medicine*, **18**, 290–304.

Ackerman, B. P., Brown, E. D. and Izard, C. E. (2004). The relations between persistent poverty and contextual risk and children's behavior in elementary school. *Developmental Psychology*, **40**, 3, 367–377.

Adams, D. and Allen, D. (2001). Assessing the need for reactive behaviour management strategies in children with learning disabilities and severe challenging behaviour. *Journal of Intellectual Disability Research*, **45**, 335–343.

Adelinis, J. D., Piazza, C. C., Fisher, W. W. and Hanley, G. P. (1997). The establishing effects of client location on self-injurious behavior. *Research in Developmental Disabilities*, **18**, 383–391.

Ahmed, Z., Fraser, W. I., Kerr, M. *et al.* (2000). The effects of reducing antipsychotic medication in people with a learning disability. *British Journal of Psychiatry*, **176**, 42–46.

Albin, R. W., Lucyshyn, J. M., Horner, R. H. and Flannery, K. B. (1996). Contextual fit for behavior support plans: a model of 'goodness of fit'. In L. K. Koegel, R. L. Koegel and G. Dunlap (eds.), *Positive Behavioral Support: Including People With Difficult Behavior in the Community*. Baltimore: Paul H. Brookes.

Allen, D. (2001). *Training Carers in Physical Interventions: Research Towards Evidence-Based Practice*. Kidderminster: BILD Publications.

Allen, D. (2008). Risk and prone restraint: reviewing the evidence. In M. Nunno, D. Day and L. Bullard (eds.). *Examining the Safety of High-Risk Interventions for Children and Young People*. New York: Child Welfare League of America.

Allen, D. and Felce, D. (1999). Service responses to challenging behaviour. In N. Bouras (ed.). *Psychiatric and Behavioural Disorders in Developmental Disabilities and Mental Retardation*. Cambridge, UK: Cambridge University Press.

Allen, D. and Harris, J. (2000). Abuse by any other name: a critique of some current approaches to behaviour management. *Mental Health Care*, **31**, 188–189.

Allen, D., McDonald, L., Dunn, C. and Doyle, A. (1997). Changing care staff approaches to the prevention and management of aggression in a residential treatment unit for persons with mental retardation and challenging behaviour. *Research in Developmental Disabilities*, **18**, 101–112.

Allen, D., Doyle, T. and Kaye, N. (2003). Plenty of gain, but no pain: a system-wide initiative. In D. Allen (ed.). *Responding to Challenging Behaviour in Persons with Intellectual Disabilities: Ethical approaches to physical intervention*. Kidderminster: British Institute of Learning Disabilities.

Allen, D., James, W., Evans, J., Hawkins, S. and Jenkins, R. (2005). Positive behavioural support: definition, current status and future directions. *Tizard Learning Disability Review*, **10**, 4–11.

Allen, D., Hawkins, S. and Cooper, V. (2006). Parents' use of physical interventions in the management of their children's challenging behaviour. *Journal of Applied Research in Intellectual Disabilities*, **19**, 356–363.

Allen, D., Lowe, K., Brophy, S. and Moore, K. (2009). Predictors of reactive strategy use in people with challenging behaviour. *Journal of Applied Research in Intellectual Disabilities*, **22**, 159–168.

Allen, D., Langthorne, P., Tonge, B. J. *et al.* (in press). Toward the prevention of behavioural and emotional difficulties in people with intellectual disabilities. *Journal of Intellectual Disabilities Research*.

Aman, M. G. (1985). Drugs in mental retardation: treatment or tragedy? *Australian and New Zealand Journal of Developmental Disabilities*, **10**, 215–226.

Aman, M. G., Singh, N. N., Stewart, A. W. and Field, C. J. (1985). The aberrant behavior checklist: a behavior rating scale for the assessment of treatment effects. *American Journal on Mental Deficiency*, **89**, 485–491.

Aman, M. G., Marks, R. E., Turbott, S. H., Wilsher, C. P. and Merry, S. N. (1991). Clinical effects of methylphenidate and thioridazine in intellectually subaverage children. *Journal of the American Academy of Child and Adolescent Psychiatry*, **30**, 246–256.

Aman, M. G., Tasse, M. J., Rojahn, J. and Hammer, D. (1996). The Nisonger CBRF: a child behavior rating form for children with developmental disabilities. *Research in Developmental Disabilities*, **17**: 1, 41–57.

Aman, M. G., De Smedt, G., Derivan, A., Lyons, B. and Findling, R. L. (2002a). Risperidone Disruptive Behavior Study Group. Double-blind, placebo-controlled study of risperidone for the treatment of disruptive behaviors in children with subaverage intelligence. *American Journal of Psychiatry*, **159**, 1337–1346.

Aman, M. G., De Smedt, G., Derivan, A., Lyons, B., Findling, R. L. and The Risperidone Disruptive Behavior Study Group (2002b). Risperidone treatment of children with disruptive behavior symptoms and subaverage IQ: a double-blind, placebo-controlled study. *American Journal of Psychiatry*, **159**, 1337–1346.

American Psychiatric Association (1994). *Diagnostic and Statistical Manual of Mental Disorders: DSM-IV*. Washington DC: American Psychiatric Association.

American Psychiatric Association (2000). *Diagnostic and Statistical Manual of Mental Disorders, 4th edition text revision*. Washington, DC: American Psychiatric Association.

Anderson, D. J., Lakin, K. C., Hill, B. K. and Chen, T. H. (1992). Social integration of older persons with Mental Retardation in residential facilities. *American Journal on Mental Retardation*, **96**, 488–501.

Anderson, J. L., Albin, R. W., Mesaros, R. A., Dunlap, G. and Morelli-Robbins, M. (1993). Issues in providing training to achieve comprehensive behavioral support. In J. Reichle and D. P. Wacker (eds.). *Communicative Alternatives to Challenging Behavior*. Baltimore: Paul H Brookes.

Asmus, J. M., Ringdahl, J. E., Sellers, J. A., Call, N. A., Andelman, M. S. and Wacker, D. P. (2004). Use of a short-term inpatient model to evaluate aberrant behavior: outcome data summaries from 1996 to 2001. *Journal of Applied Behavior Analysis*, **37**, 283–304.

Azrin, N. H. and Foxx, R. M. (1971). A rapid method of toilet training the institutionalized retarded. *Journal of Applied Behavior Analysis*, **4**, 89–99.

Azrin, N. H., Besalal, V. A., Jamner, J. P. and Caputo, J. N. (1988). Comparative study of behavioral methods of treating severe self-injury. *Behavioral Residential Treatment*, **3**, 119–152.

Baer, D. M., Wolf, M. M. and Risley, T. R. (1968). Some current dimensions of applied behavior analysis. *Journal of Applied Behavior Analysis*, **1**, 91–97.

Baer, D. M., Wolf, M. M. and Risley, T. R. (1987). Some still current dimensions of applied behavior analysis. *Journal of Applied Behavior Analysis*, **20**, 313–327.

Bailey, J. S. and Meyerson, L. (1969). Vibration as a reinforcer with a profoundly retarded child. *Journal of Applied Behavior Analysis*, **2**, 135–137.

Baird, G., Simonoff, E., Pickles, A. *et al.* (2006). Prevalence of disorders of the autism spectrum in a population cohort of children in South Thames: the Special Needs and Autism Project (SNAP). *Lancet*, **368**, 210–215.

Baker, B. L., Blacher, J., Crnic, K. and Edelbrock, C. (2002). Behavior problems and parenting stress in families of three-year-old children with and without developmental delays. *American Journal on Mental Retardation*, **107**, 433–444.

Baker, P. and Allen, D. (2001). Physical abuse and physical interventions in learning disabilities: an element of risk? *Journal of Adult Protection*, **3**, 25–31.

Ball, T., Bush, A. and Emerson, E. (2004). *Psychological Interventions for Severely Challenging Behaviours Shown by People with Learning Disabilities*. Leicester: British Psychological Society.

Bannerman, D. J., Sheldon, J. B., Sherman, J. A. and Harchik, A. E. (1990). Balancing the right to habilitation with the right to personal liberties: the rights of people with developmental disabilities to eat too many doughnuts and take a nap. *Journal of Applied Behavior Analysis*, **23**, 79–89.

Barkham, M. and Mellor-Clark, J. (2003). Bridging evidence-based practice and practice-based evidence: developing a rigorous and relevant knowledge for the psychological therapies. *Clinical Psychology and Psychotherapy*, **10**, 319–327.

Barlow, D. H., Nock, M. K. and Hersen, M. (2008). *Single Case Experimental Designs: Strategies for Studying Behavior Change*. Boston: Allyn & Bacon.

Beadle-Brown, J., Murphy, G. and Wing, L. (2005). Long-term outcome for people with severe intellectual disabilities: impact of social impairment. *American Journal on Mental Retardation*, **110**, 1–12.

Beail, N. and Warden, S. (1995). Sexual abuse of adults with learning disabilities. *Journal of Intellectual Disability Research* **39**, 382–387.

Beasley, C., Dellva, M., Tamura, R. *et al.* (1999). Randomised double-blind comparison of the incidence of tardive dyskinesia in patients with schizophrenia during long-term treatment with olanzapine or haloperidol. *British Journal of Psychiatry*, **174**: 1, 23–30.

Beaudet, A. L. (2007). Autism: highly heritable but not inherited. *Nature Medicine*, **13**, 534–536.

Bellugi, U., Lichtenberger, L., Mills, D., Galaburda, A. and Korenberg, J. R. (1999). Bridging cognition, the brain and molecular genetics: Evidence from Williams syndrome. *Trends in Neurosciences*, **22**, 197–207.

Benazzi, F. (1998). Risperidone-induced hepatotoxicity. *Pharmacopsychiatry*, **31**, 241.

Bergk, J., Einsiedler, B. and Steinert, T. (2008). Feasibility of randomized controlled trails on seclusion and mechanical restraint. *Clinical Trials*, **5**, 356–363.

Bergstrom, N. (2008). The gap between discovery and practice implementation in evidence-based practice: is practice-based evidence a solution? *International Journal of Evidence-Based Healthcare*, **6**, 135–136.

Berkson, G. (1983). Repetitive stereotyped behaviors. *American Journal on Mental Deficiency*, **88**, 239–246.

Berkson, G. and Tupa, M. (2000). Early development of stereotyped and self-injurious behaviors. *Journal of Early Intervention*, **23**, 1–19.

Biersdorff, K. K. (1991). Pain insensitivity and indifference: alternate explanations for some medical catastrophes. *Mental Retardation*, **29**, 359–362.

Biersdorff, K. K. (1994). Incidence if significantly altered pain experience among individuals with developmental disabilities. *American Journal on Mental Retardation*, **98**, 619–631.

Bihm, E. M., Kienlen, T. L., Ness, M. E. and Poindexter, A. R. (1991). Factor structure of the Motivation Assessment Scale for persons with mental retardation. *Psychological Reports*, **68**, 1235–1238.

Bijou, S. W. (1966). A functional analysis of retarded development. In N. Ellis (ed.), *International Review of Research in Mental Retardation, Volume 1*, New York: Academic Press.

Bijou, S. W. and Baer, D. M. (1978). *Behavior Analysis of Child Development*. Englewood Cliffs, NJ: Prentice Hall.

Bird, F., Dores, P. A., Moniz, D. and Robinson, J. (1989). Reducing severe aggressive and self-injurious behaviours with functional communication training. *American Journal on Mental Retardation*, **94**, 37–48.

Black, L., Cullen, C. and Novaco, R. (1997). Anger assessment for people with mild learning disabilities in secure settings. In B. S. Kroese, D. Dagnan and K. Loumidis, eds. *Cognitive-Behaviour Therapy for People with Learning Disabilities*. London: Routledge.

Blackburn, R. (2006). Physical interventions and autism: a service user's perspective. In S. Paley and J. Brooke (eds.), *Good Practice in Physical Interventions*. Kidderminster: British Institute of Learning Disabilities.

Blunden, R. and Allen, D. (1987). *Facing the Challenge: An Ordinary Life for People with Learning Difficulties and Challenging Behaviours*. London: King's Fund.

Boisjoli, R., Vitaro, F., Lacourse, E., Barker, E. D. and Tremblay, R. E. (2007). Impact and clinical significance of a preventative intervention for disruptive boys: 15 year follow up. *British Journal of Psychiatry*, **191**, 415–419.

Bonell-Pascual, E., Huline-Dickens, S., Hollins, S., Esterhuyzen, A., Sedgwick, P. and Abdelnoor, A. (1999). Bereavement and grief in adults with learning disabilities: a follow-up study. *British Journal of Psychiatry*, **175**, 348–350.

Bornstein, M. and Bradley, R. H. (2003). *Socioeconomic Status, Parenting, and Child Development*. Mahwah, NJ: Lawrence Erlbaum Associates.

Borrero, C. S. W. and Borrero, J. C. (2008). Descriptive and experimental analyses of potential precursors to problem behavior. *Journal of Applied Behavior Analysis*, **41**, 83–96.

Borthwick Duffy S. A. (1994). Prevalence of destructive behaviors. In T. Thompson and D. B. Gray (eds.). *Destructive Behavior in Developmental Disabilities: Diagnosis and Treatment*, Thousand Oaks: Sage.

Bosch, J., Van Dyke, C., Smith, S. M. and Poulton, S. (1997). Role of medical conditions in the exacerbation of self-injurious behavior: an exploratory study. *Mental Retardation*, **35**: 2, 124–130.

Bowie, V. (1996). *Coping with Violence. A Guide for the Human Services*. London: Whiting & Birch.

Boyd, R. D. (1993). Antipsychotic malignant syndrome and mental retardation: review and analysis of 29 cases. *American Journal of Mental Retardation*, **98**: 1, 143–155.

Bradley, R. H. and Corwyn, R. F. (2002). Socioeconomic status and child development. *Annual Review of Psychology*, **53**, 371–399.

Bradley, R. H., Corwyn, R. F., McAdoo, H. P. and Garcia, C. C. (2001). The home environments of children in the United States: part I. Variations by age, ethnicity, and poverty status. *Child Development*, **72**, 1844–1867.

Bradshaw, J. (2001). *Poverty: The Outcomes for Children*. London: Family Policy Studies Centre.

Breau, L. M., Camfield, C. S., McGrath, P. J. and Finley, G. A. (2007). Pain's impact on adaptive functioning. *Journal of Intellectual Disability Research*, **51**: Pt 2, 125–134.

Brereton, A. V., Tonge, B. J. and Einfeld, S. L. (2006). Psychopathology in children and adolescents with autism compared to young people with intellectual disability. *Journal of Autism & Developmental Disorders*, **36**, 863–870.

British Institute of Learning Disabilities (2006). *Code of Practice for the Use of Physical Interventions. A Guide for Trainers and Commissioners of Training*. 2nd edn, Kidderminster: BILD Publications.

Broberg, M., Blacher, J. and Emerson, E. (2009). Editorial: Resilience. *Journal of Intellectual Disability Research*, **53**, 955–956.

Broidy, L. M., Nagin, D. S., Tremblay, R. E., Bates, J. E., Brame, B. and Dodge, K. (2003). Developmental trajectories of childhood disruptive behaviours and adolescent delinquency: a six site, cross national study. *Developmental Psychology*, **39**, 222–245.

Bromley, J. and Emerson, E. (1995). Beliefs and emotional reactions of care staff working with people with challenging behaviour. *Journal of Intellectual Disability Research*, **39**, 341–352.

Brooks-Gunn, J. and Duncan, G. (1997). The effects of poverty on children and youth. *The Future of Children*, **7**, 55–71.

Browder, D. M. (1991). *Assessment of Individuals with Severe Disabilities*. Baltimore: Brookes.

Browder, D. M. (2001). *Curriculum and Assessment for Students with Moderate and Severe Disabilities*. New York: Guilford Press.

Brylewski, J. and Wiggs, L. (1999). Sleep problems and daytime challenging behaviour in a community-based sample of adults with intellectual disability. *Journal of Intellectual Disability Research*, **43**, 504–512.

Bull, M. and Vecchio, F. (1978). Behavior therapy for a child with Lesch–Nyhan syndrome. *Developmental Medicine and Child Neurology*, **20**, 368–375.

Bullard, L., Fulmore, D. and Johnson, K. (2003). *Reducing the Use of Restraint and Seclusion. Promising Practices and Successful Strategies.* Washington: CWLA Press.

Burchardt, T. and Huerta, M. C. (2008). Introduction: resilience and social exclusion. *Social Policy and Society*, **8**, 59–61.

Burger, K. (2010). How does early childhood care and education affect cognitive development? An international review of the effects of early interventions for children from different social backgrounds. *Early Childhood Research Quarterly*, **25**, 140–165.

Buss, A. H. and Plomin, R. (1984). *Temperament: Early Developing Personality Traits.* Hillsdale: Lawrence Erlbaum.

Buzan, R. D., Dubovsky, S. L., Firestone, D. and Dal Pozzo, E. (1998). Use of clozapine in 10 mentally retarded adults. *Journal of Neuropsychiatry and Clinical Neurosciences*, **10**, 93–95.

Cairns, R. B., Cairns, B. D., Neckerman, H. J., Ferguson, L. L. and Gariépy, J. L. (1989). Growth and aggression, 1: Childhood to early adolescence. *Developmental Psychology*, **25**, 320–330.

Cambridge, P. (1999). The First Hit: a case study of the physical abuse of people with learning disabilities and challenging behaviour in a residential service. *Disability and Society*, **14**, 285–308.

Cameron, M. J., Maguire, R. W. and Maguire, M. (1998). Lifeway influences on challenging behaviors. In J. K. Luiselli and M. J. Cameron, eds. *Antecedent Control: Innovative Approaches to Behavioral Support.* Baltimore: Paul H. Brookes.

Camp, E. M., Iwata, B. A., Hammond, J. L. and Bloom, S. E. (2009). Antecedent versus consequent events as predictors of problem behavior. *Journal of Applied Behavior Analysis*, **42**, 469–483.

Campbell, J. (2003). Efficacy of behavioral interventions for reducing problem behaviors in persons with autism: a quantitative synthesis of single-subject research. *Research in Developmental Disabilities*, **24**, 120–138.

Campbell, M., Armenteros, J. L., Malone, R. P., Adams, P. B., Eisenberg, Z. W. and Overall, J. E. (1997). Antipsychotic-related dyskinesias in autistic children: a prospective, longitudinal study. *Journal of the American Academy of Child and Adolescent Psychiatry*, **36**, 835–843.

Caplan, G. (1964). *Principles of Preventative Psychology.* New York, NY: Basic Books.

Carmeli, E., Orbach, I., Zinger-Vaknin, T., Morad, M. and Merrick, J. (2008). Physical training and well-being in older adults with mild intellectual disability: a residential care study. *Journal of Applied Research in Intellectual Disabilities*, **21**, 457–465.

Carr, E. G. (1977). The motivation of self injurious behavior: a review of some hypotheses. *Psychological Bulletin*, **84**, 800–816.

Carr, E. G. (1988). Functional equivalence as a mechanism of response generalization. In R. H. Horner, G. Dunlap and R. L. Koegel, eds. *Generalization and Maintenance: Life Style Changes in Applied Settings.* Baltimore: Brookes.

Carr, E. G. (2007). The expanding vision of positive behavior support: Research perspectives on happiness, helpfulness, hopefulness. *Journal of Positive Behavior Interventions*, **9**, 3–14.

Carr, E. G. and Durand, V. M. (1985a). Reducing behavior problems through functional communication training. *Journal of Applied Behavior Analysis*, **18**, 111–126.

Carr, E. G. and Durand, V. M. (1985b). The social communicative basis of severe behavior problems in children. In S. Reiss and R. R. Bootzin, eds., *Theoretical Issues in Behavior Therapy*. New York: Academic Press.

Carr, E. G. and Newsom, C. D. (1985). Demand-related tantrums: Conceptualization and treatment. *Behavior Modification*, **9**, 403–426.

Carr, E. G. and Carlson, J. I. (1993). Reduction of severe behavior problems in the community using a multicomponent treatment approach. *Journal of Applied Behavior Analysis*, **26**, 157–172.

Carr, E. G. and Smith, C. E. (1995). Biological setting events for self-injury. *Mental Retardation and Developmental Disabilities Research Reviews*, **1**, 94–98.

Carr, E. G., Newsom, C. D. and Binkoff, J. (1976). Stimulus control of self destructive behavior in a psychotic child. *Journal of Abnormal Child Psychology*, **4**, 139–153.

Carr, E. G., Robinson, S. and Palumbo, L. W. (1990a). The wrong issue: aversive versus nonaversive treatment. The right issue: functional versus nonfunctional treatment. In A. C. Repp and N. N. Singh, eds. *Current Perspectives in the Use of Nonaversive and Aversive Interventions with Developmentally Disabled Persons*. Sycamore, IL: Sycamore Press.

Carr, E. G., Robinson, S., Taylor, J. C. and Carlson, J. I. (1990b). *Positive Approaches to the Treatment of Severe Behavior Problems in Persons with Developmental Disabilities*. Seattle: The Association for Persons with Severe Handicaps.

Carr, E. G., Taylor, J. C. and Robinson, S. (1991). The effects of severe behavior problems in children on the teaching behavior of adults. *Journal of Applied Behavior Analysis*, **24**, 523–535.

Carr, E. G., Levin, L., McConnachie, G., Carlson, J. I., Kemp, D. C. and Smith, C. E. (1994). *Communication-Based Intervention for Problem Behavior: A User's Guide for Producing Positive Change*. Baltimore: Brookes.

Carr, E. G., Reeve, C. E. and Magito-McLaughlin, D. (1996). Contextual influences on problem behavior in people with developmental disabilities. In L. K. Koegel, R. L. Koegel and G. Dunlap, eds. *Positive Behavioral Support: Including People With Difficult Behavior in the Community*. Baltimore: Paul H. Brookes.

Carr, E. G., Yarbrough, S. C. and Langdon, N. A. (1997). Effects of idiosyncratic stimulus variables on functional analysis outcomes. *Journal of Applied Behavior Analysis*, **30**, 673–686.

Carr, E. G., Carlson, J. I., Langdon, N. A., Magito-McLaughlin, D. and Yarbrough, S. C. (1998). Two perspectives on antecedent control: Molecular and molar. In J. K. Luiselli and M. J. Cameron, eds., *Antecedent Control: Innovative Approaches to Behavioral Support*. Baltimore: Paul H. Brookes.

Carr, E. G., Horner, R. H., Turnbull, A. P. *et al.* (1999). *Positive Behavior Support For People with Developmental Disabilities*. Washington, DC: American Association on Mental Retardation.

Carr, E. G., Dunlap, G., Horner, R. H. *et al.* (2002). Positive behavior support: evolution of an applied science. *Journal of Positive Behavior Interventions*, **4**, 4–16.

Carr, E. G., Ladd, M. V. and Schulte, C. F. (2008). Validation of the Contextual Assessment Inventory for problem behavior. *Journal of Positive Behavior Interventions*, **10**, 91–104.

Carr, J. E. and LeBlanc, L. A. (2006). Noncontingent reinforcement as antecedent behavior support. In J. K. Luiselli, ed. *Antecedent Assessment and Intervention*, Baltimore: Paul H. Brookes.

Cataldo, M. F. (1991). The effects of punishment and other behavior reducing procedures on the destructive behaviors of persons with developmental disabilities. In National Institute of Health, ed. *Treatment of Destructive Behaviors in Persons with Developmental Disabilities*. Washington: Department of Health and Human Services.

Cautela, J. R. and Groden, J. (1978). *Relaxation. A Comprehensive Manual for Adults, Children, and Children with Special Needs*. Illinois: Research Press Company.

Chadwick, O., Kusel, Y., Cuddy, M. and Taylor, E. (2005). Psychiatric diagnoses and behaviour problems from childhood to early adolescence in young people with severe intellectual disabilities. *Psychological Medicine*, **35**, 751–760.

Chadwick, O., Kusel, Y. and Cuddy, M. (2008). Factors associated with the risk of behaviour problems in adolescents with severe intellectual disabilities. *Journal of Intellectual Disability Research*, **52**, 864–876.

Chapman, D., Scott, K. and Stanton-Chapman, T. (2008). Public health approach to the study of mental retardation. *American Journal on Mental Retardation*, **113**, 102–116.

Charlot, L. R. and Mikklesen, E. J. (2006). Commonly employed psychopathology instruments for individuals with intellectual disabilities. In J. Hogg and A. Langa, eds. *Assessing Adults with Intellectual Disabilities: A Service Providers' Guide*. Oxford: Blackwell.

Chasson, G., Harris, G. and Neely, W. (2007). Cost comparison of early intensive behavioral intervention and special education for children with autism. *Journal of Child and Family Studies*, **16**, 401–413.

Chen, D., Downing, J. E. and Peckham-Hardin, K. D. (2002). Working with families of diverse cultural and linguistic backgrounds: considerations for culturally responsive positive behavior supports. In J. M. Lucyshyn, G. Dunlap and R. W. Albin, eds. *Families and Positive Behavior Support*. Baltimore: Brookes.

Child Welfare League of America (2004). *CWLA Best Practice Guidelines*. Washington DC: CWLA.

Churchill, H. and Clarke, K. (2009). Investing in parenting education: a critical review of policy and provision in England. *Social Policy and Society*, **9**, 39–53.

Clarke, D. J. (1989). Antilibidinal drugs and mental retardation: a review. *Medicine, Science and the Law*, **29**: 2, 136–146.

Clements, J. and Zarkowska, E. (2000). *Behavioural Concerns and Autistic Spectrum Disorders*. London: Jessica Kingsley.

Cochrane, A. L. (1972). *Effectiveness and Efficiency: Random Reflection on Health Services*. London: Nuffield Provincial Hospitals Trust.

Coe, D. A., Matson, J. L., Russell, D. W., Slifer, K. J., Capone, G. and Baglio, C. (1999). Behavior problems of children with Down syndrome and life events. *Journal of Autism and Developmental Disorders*, **29**, 149–156.

Coie, J. D., Miller-Johnson, S. and Bagwell, C. (2000). Prevention science. In A. Sameroff, M. Lewis and S. Miller, eds. *Handbook of Developmental Psychopathology*. New York: Plenum.

Coleman, J. and Hagell, A. (2007). *Adolescent Risk and Resilience: Against the Odds*. Chichester: Wiley.

Colton, D. (2008). Leadership's and program's role in organizational and cultural change to reduce seclusion and restraints. In M. Nunno, D. Day and L. Bullard, eds. *Examining the Safety of High-risk Interventions for Children and Young people*. New York: Child Welfare League of America.

Conger, R. D. and Conger, K. J. (2002). Resilience in Midwestern families: selected findings from the first decade of a prospective, longitudinal study. *Journal of Marriage & Family*, **64**, 361–373.

Conger, R. D. and Donnellan, M. B. (2007). An interactionist perspective on the socioeconomic context of human development. *Annual Review of Psychology*, **58**, 175–199.

Conger, R. D., Conger, K. J., Elder, G. H., Lorenz, F. C., Simons, R. L. and Whitbeck, L. B. (1992). A family process model of economic hardship and adjustment of early adolescent boys. *Child Development*, **3**, 526–554.

Cooper, J., Heron, T. and Heward, W. (2006). *Applied Behavior Analysis*. New York: Prentice-Hall.

Cooper, L. J., Wacker, D. P., Thursby, D. *et al.* (1992). Analysis of the effects of task preferences, task demands and adult attention on child behavior in outpatient and classroom setting. *Journal of Applied Behavior Analysis*, **25**, 823–840.

Cooper, S. A., Smiley, E., Finlayson, J. *et al.* (2007). The prevalence, incidence and factors predictive of mental ill-health in adults with profound intellectual disabilities. *Journal of Applied Research in Intellectual Disabilities*, **20**, 493–501.

Cooper, S. A., Smiley, E., Allan, L. *et al.* (2009a). Adults with intellectual disabilities: prevalence, incidence and remission of self-injurious behaviour and related factors. *Journal of Intellectual Disability Research*, **53**, 200–216.

Cooper, S. A., Smiley, E., Jackson, A. *et al.* (2009b). Adults with intellectual disabilities: prevalence, incidence and remission of aggressive behaviour and related factors. *Journal of Intellectual Disability Research*, **53**, 217–232.

Costello, E. J., Compton, S. N., Keeler, G. and Angold, A. (2003). Relationships between poverty and psychopathology: a natural experiment. *JAMA*, **290**, 2023–2029.

Cottle, M., Kuipers, L., Murphy, G. and Oakes, P. (1995). Expressed emotion: attributions and coping in staff who have been victims of violent incidents. *Mental Handicap Research*, **8**, 168–183.

Cox, A. and Rutter, M. (1985). Diagnostic appraisal and interviewing. In M. Rutter and L. Hersov, eds. *Child and Adolescent Psychiatry: Modern Approaches*, Oxford: Blackwell Scientific.

Crocker, A. G., Mercier, C., Lachapelle, Y., Brunet, A., Morin, D. and Roy, M. E. (2006). Prevalence and types of aggressive behaviour among adults with intellectual disabilities. *Journal of Intellectual Disability Research*, **50**, 652–661.

Crosland, K. A., Cigales, M., Dunlap, G. *et al.* (2008). Using staff training to decrease restrictive procedures at two facilities for foster care children. *Research on Social Work in Practice*, **18**, 401–409.

Cullen, C., Hattersley, J. and Tennant, L. (1981). Establishing behaviour: the constructional approach. In G. Davey, ed. *Applications of Conditioning Theory*. London: Methuen.

Cummings, E. M., Iannotti, R. J. and Zahn-Waxler, C. (1989). Aggression between peers in early childhood: Individual continuity and developmental change. *Child Development*, **60**, 887–895.

Cunningham, J., McDonnell, A., Easton, S. and Sturmey, P. (2003). Social validation data on three methods of physical restraint: views of consumers, staff and students. *Research in Developmental Disabilities*, **24**, 307–316.

Dagnan, D. and Weston, C. (2006). Physical intervention with people with intellectual disabilities: The influence of cognitive and emotional variables. *Journal of Applied Research in Intellectual Disabilities*, **19**, 219–222.

Dagnan, D., Jahoda, A. and Kroese, B. S. (2007). Cognitive behaviour therapy. In A. Carr, G. O'Reilly, P. N. Walsh and J. McEvoy (eds.). *The Handbook of Intellectual Disability and Clinical Psychology Practice*. London: Routledge.

Davidson, P. W., Cain, N. N., Sloane-Reeves, J. E. *et al.* (1994). Characteristics of community based individuals with mental retardation and aggressive behavioral disorders. *American Journal on Mental Retardation*, **98**, 704–716.

Davis, C. A., Brady, M. P., Williams, R. E. and Hamilton, R. (1992). Effects of high-probability requests on the acquisition and generalization and responses to requests in young children with behavior disorders. *Journal of Applied Behavior Analysis*, **25**, 905–916.

Davis, S., Wehmeyer, M. L., Board, J. P., Fox, S., Maher, F. and Roberts, B. (1998). Interdisciplinary teams. In S. Reiss and M. G. Aman, eds. *Psychotropic Medication and Developmental Disabilities: The International Consensus Handbook*. Ohio: Nisonger Center, Ohio State University.

Davis-Kean, P. E. (2005). The influence of parent education and family income on child achievement: the indirect role of parental expectations and the home environment. *Journal of Family Psychology*, **19**, 294–304.

de Graaf, I., Speetjens, P., Smit, F., de Wolff, M. and Tavecchio, L. (2008a). Effectiveness of the triple p positive parenting program on behavioral problems in children: a meta-analysis. *Behavior Modification*, **32**, 714–735.

de Graaf, I., Speetjens, P., Smit, F., de Wolff, M. and Tavecchio, L. (2008b). Effectiveness of the triple p positive parenting program on parenting: a meta-analysis. *Family Relations*, **57**, 553–566.

de Leon, J., Greenlee, B., Barber, J., Sabaawi, M. and Singh, N. N. (2009). Practical guidelines for the use of new generation anti-psychotic drugs (except clozapine) in adult individuals with intellectual disabilities. *Research in Developmental Disabilities*, **30**, 613–669.

de Lissovoy, V. (1962). Head banging in early childhood. *Child Development*, **33**, 43–56.

de Lissovoy, V. (1963). Head banging in early childhood: a suggested cause. *Journal of Genetic Psychology*, **102**, 109–114.

Deb, S., Thomas, M. and Bright, C. (2001). Mental disorder in adults with intellectual disability. 1: Prevalence of functional psychiatric illness among a community-based population aged between 16 and 64 years. *Journal of Intellectual Disability Research*, **45**, 495–505.

Deb, S., Clarke, D. and Unwin, G. (2006). *Using Medication to Manage Behaviour Problems Among Adults with a Learning Disability: Quick Reference Guide*. London: Mencap.

Deb, S., Sohanpal, S. K., Soni, R., Lenôtre, L. and Unwin, G. (2007). The effectiveness of antipsychotic medication in the management of behaviour problems in adults with intellectual disabilities. *Journal of Intellectual Disability Research*, 51, 766–777.

Deb, S., Chaplin, R., Sohanpal, S., Unwin, G., Soni, R. and Lenotre, L. (2008). The effectiveness of mood stabilizers and antiepileptic medication for the management of behaviour problems in adults with intellectual disability: a systematic review. *Journal of Intellectual Disability Research*, 52, 107–113.

Dekker, M. C. and Koot, H. M. (2003). DSM-IV disorders in children with borderline to moderate intellectual disability. II: Child and family factors. *Journal of the American Academy of Child and Adolescent Psychiatry*, 42, 923–931.

DeLeon, I. G. and Iwata, B. A. (1996). Evaluation of a multiple stimulus presentation format for assessing reinforcer preferences. *Journal of Applied Behavior Analysis*, 29, 519–533.

Demchak, M. A. and Bossert, K. W. (1996). *Assessing Problem Behaviors*. Washington, DC: American Association on Intellectual and Developmental Disabilities.

Department of Health (1993). *Services for People with Learning Disabilities and Challenging Behaviour or Mental Health Needs*. London Department of Health.

Department of Health (2007). *Services for People with Learning Disabilities and Challenging Behaviour or Mental Health Needs*: (Revised Edition). London: Department of Health.

Department of Health and Department for Education and Skills (2002). *Guidance for Restrictive Physical Interventions. How to provide safe services for people with Learning Disabilities and Autistic Spectrum Disorder*. London: Department of Health

Department of Human Services (2009). *Physical Restraint in Disability Services*. Melbourne: Office of the Senior Practitioner.

Derby, K. M., Wacker, D. P., Sasso, G. *et al.* (1992). Brief functional assessment techniques to evaluate aberrant behavior in an outpatient setting: A summary of 79 cases. *Journal of Applied Behavior Analysis*, 25, 713–721.

Derby, K. M., Wacker, D. P., Peck, S. *et al.* (1994). Functional analysis of separate topographies of aberrant behavior. *Journal of Applied Behavior Analysis*, 27, 267–278.

Derby, K. M., Fisher, W. W., Piazza, C. C. and Wilke, A. E. (1998). The effects of non-contingent and contingent attention for self-injury, manding and collateral responses. *Behavior Modification*, 22, 474–484.

Desrochers, M. N., Hile, M. G. and Williams-Moseley, T. L. (1997). Survey of functional assessment procedures used with individuals who display mental retardation and severe problem behaviors. *American Journal on Mental Retardation*, 101, 535–546.

Deveau, R. and McGill, P. (2009). Physical interventions for adults with intellectual disabilities: survey of use, policy, training and monitoring. *Journal of Applied Research in Intellectual Disabilities*, 22, 152–158.

Di Terlizzi, M., Cambridge, P. and Maras, P. (1999). Gender, ethnicity and challenging behaviour: a literature review and exploratory study. *Tizard Learning Disability Review*, 4, 33–44.

Dickinson, H., Parkinson, K., Ravens-Sieberer, U. *et al.* (2007). Self-reported quality of life of 8–12-year-old children with cerebral palsy: a crosssectional European study. *Lancet*, 369, 2171–2178.

Didden, R., Duker, P. C. and Korzilius, H. (1997). Meta-analytic study on treatment effectiveness for problem behaviors with individuals who have mental retardation. *American Journal of Mental Retardation*, 101, 387–399.

Didden, R., Korzilius, H., van Oorsouw, W. and Sturmey, P. (2006). Behavioral treatment of challenging behaviors in individuals with mild mental retardation: meta-analysis of single-subject research. *American Journal on Mental Retardation*, **111**, 290–298.

Dishion, T. J., Shaw, D., Connell, A., Gardner, F., Weaver, C. and Wilson, M. (2008). The Family Check-Up with high-risk indigent families: Preventing problem behavior by increasing parents' positive behavior support in early childhood. *Child Development*, **79**, 1395–1414.

Dixon, D. R., Kurtz, P. F. and Chin, M. D. (2008). A systematic review of challenging behaviors in children exposed prenatally to substances of abuse. *Research in Developmental Disabilities*, **29**, 483–502.

Donnellan, A. M., Mirenda, P., Mesaros, R. and Fassbender, L. (1984). Analyzing the communicative functions of aberrant behavior. *Journal of the Association for Persons with Severe Handicaps*, **9**, 201–212.

Donnellan, A. M., LaVigna, G. W., Negri Shoultz, N. and Fassbender, L. L. (1988). *Progress Without Punishment: Effective Approaches for Learners with Behavior Problems*. New York: Teachers College Press.

Dossetor, D. R., Couryer, S. and Nicol, A. R. (1991). Massage for very severe self-injurious behaviour in a girl with Cornelia de Lange syndrome. *Developmental Medicine and Child Neurology*, **33**, 636–644.

Doyle, O., Harmon, C. P., Heckman, J. J. and Tremblay, R. E. (2009). Investing in early human development: timing and economic efficiency. *Economics and Human Biology*, **7**, 1–6.

Duker, P. C. and Rasing, E. (1989). Effects of redesigning the physical environment on self stimulation and on task behavior in three autistic type developmentally disabled individuals. *Journal of Autism and Developmental Disorders*, **19**, 449–460.

Duker, P. C. and Sigafoos, J. (1998). The Motivation Assessment Scale: reliability and construct validity across three topographies of behavior. *Research in Developmental Disabilities*, **19**, 131–141.

Duncan, D., Matson, J. L., Bamburg, J. W., Cherry, K. E. and Buckley, T. (1999). The relationship of self-injurious behavior and aggression to social skills in persons with severe and profound learning disability. *Research in Developmental Disabilities*, **20**, 441–448.

Duncan, G. J. and Brooks-Gunn, J. (2000). Family poverty, welfare reform, and child development. *Child Development*, **71**, 188–196.

Dunlap, G., dePerczel, M., Clarke, S. *et al.* (1994). Choice making to promote adaptive behavior for students with emotional and behavioral challenges. *Journal of Applied Behavior Analysis*, **27**, 505–518.

Dunlap, G., Foster-Johnson, L., Clarke, S., Kern, L. and Childs, K. E. (1995). Modifying activities to produce functional outcomes: Effects on the problem behaviors of students with disabilities. *Journal of the Association For Persons With Severe Handicaps*, **20**, 248–258.

Dunlap, G., Clarke, S. and Steiner, M. (1999). Intervention research in behavioral and developmental disabilities: 1980–1997. *Journal of Positive Behavior Interventions*, **1**, 170–180.

Durand, V.M. (1986). Self injurious behavior as intentional communication. In K.D. Gadow, ed., *Advances in Learning and Behavioral Disabilities*. London: JAI Press.

Durand, V.M. (1990). *Severe Behavior Problems: A Functional Communication Training Approach*. New York: Guilford Press.

Durand, V.M. (1999). Functional communication training using assistive devices: recruiting natural communities of reinforcement. *Journal of Applied Behavior Analysis*, **32**, 247–267.

Durand, V.M. and Crimmins, D.B. (1988). Identifying the variables maintaining self injurious behavior. *Journal of Autism and Developmental Disorders*, **18**, 99–115.

Durand, V.M. and Crimmins, D.B. (1992). *The Motivation Assessment Scale*. Topkepa, KS: Monaco & Associates.

Durand, V.M. and Mapstone, E. (1998). Influence of mood inducing music on challenging behavior. *American Journal of Mental Retardation*, **102**, 367–378.

Durand, V.M., Crimmins, D., Caulfield, M. and Taylor, J. (1989). Reinforcer assessment I: Using problem behavior to select reinforcers. *Journal of the Association for Persons with Severe Handicaps*, **14**, 113–126.

Durand, V.M., Berotti, D. and Weiner, J.S. (1993). Functional communication training: factors affecting effectiveness, generalization and maintenance. In J. Reichle and D.P. Wacker, eds. *Communicative Alternatives to Challenging Behavior*. Baltimore: Brookes.

Durand, V.M., Gernert-Dott, P. and Mapstone, E. (1996). Treatment of sleep disorders in children with developmental disabilities. *Journal of the Association For Persons With Severe Handicaps*, **21**, 114–122.

Durkin, M. (2002). The epidemiology of developmental disabilities in low-income countries. *Mental Retardation and Developmental Disabilities Research Reviews*, **8**: 3, 206–211.

Durlak, J.A. and Wells, A.M. (1998). Evaluation of indicated preventive intervention (secondary prevention) mental health programs for children and adolescents. *American Journal of Community Psychology*, **26**, 775–802.

Dyer, K. and Larsson, E.V. (1997). Developing functional communication skills: alternatives to severe behavior disorders. In N.N. Singh, ed. *Prevention and Treatment of Severe Behavior Problems: Models and Methods in Developmental Disabilities*. Baltimore: Brookes.

Dyer, K., Dunlap, G. and Winterling, V. (1990). Effects of choice making on the serious problem behaviors of students with severe handicaps. *Journal of Applied Behavior Analysis*, **23**, 515–524.

Dykens, E.M. (2003). Anxiety, fears, and phobias in persons with Williams syndrome. *Developmental Neuropsychology*, **23**, 291–316.

Dykens, E.M. and Cohen, D.L. (1996). Effects of Special Olympics International on social competence in persons with mental retardation. *Journal of the American Academy of Child and Adolescent Psychiatry*, **35**, 223–229.

Dykens, E.M., Hodapp, R.M. and Finucane, B.M. (2000). *Genetics and Mental Retardation Syndromes: A New Look at Behavior and Interventions*. Baltimore: Paul H. Brookes Publishing.

Dykens, E. M., Rosner, B. A. and Ly, T. M. (2001). Drawings by individuals with Williams syndrome: are people different from shapes? *American Journal of Mental Retardation*, **106**, 94–107.

Edelson, S. M., Taubman, M. T. and Lovaas, O. I. (1983). Some social contexts of self destructive behavior. *Journal of Abnormal Child Psychology*, **11**, 299–312.

Edwards, R. (1999a). Physical restraint and gender: whose role is it anyway? *Learning Disability Practice*, **2**, 12–15.

Edwards, R. (1999b). The laying on of hands: nursing staff talk about physical restraint. *Journal of Learning Disabilities for Nursing, Health and Social Care*, **3**, 136–143.

Einfeld, S. and Tonge, B. J. (2002). *Manual for the Developmental Behaviour Checklist*, 2nd edn, Clayton, AUS: Centre for Developmental Psychiatry, Monash University.

Einfeld, S. and Emerson, E. (2008). Intellectual disability. In M. Rutter, D. Bishop, D. Pine *et al.* eds. *Rutter's Child and Adolescent Psychiatry*. Oxford: Blackwell.

Einfeld, S., Tonge, B. and Turner, G. (1999a). Longitudinal course of behavioral and emotional problems in fragile X syndrome. *American Journal of Medical Genetics*, **87**, 436–439.

Einfeld, S., Piccinin, A., Mackinnon, A. *et al.* (2006). Psychopathology in young people with intellectual disability. *Journal of the American Medical Association*, **296**: 16, 1981–1989.

Einfeld, S., Stancliffe, R., Gray, K., Sofronoff, K., Emerson, E. and Yasamy, M. T. (2009). Interventions provided by parents for children with intellectual disabilities in low and middle income countries. Sydney: Australian Family & Disability Studies Research Collaboration, University of Sydney.

Einfeld, S. L. (1990). Guidelines for the use of psychotropic medication in patients with intellectual handicaps. *Australian and New Zealand Journal of Developmental Disabilities*, **16**, 71–73.

Einfeld, S. L. (1992). Clinical assessment of psychiatric symptoms in mentally retarded individuals. *Australian New Zealand Journal of Psychiatry*, **26**, 48–63.

Einfeld, S. L. (2005). Behaviour problems in children with genetic disorders causing intellectual disability. *Educational Psychology*, **25**: 2–3, 341–346

Einfeld, S. L. and Tonge, B. J. (1995). The Developmental Behavior Checklist: the development and validation of an instrument to assess behavioral and emotional disturbance in children and adolescents with mental retardation. *Journal of Autism and Developmental Disorders* **25**, 81–104.

Einfeld, S. L., Smith, A., Durvasula, S., Florio, T. and Tonge, B. J. (1999b). Behavior and emotional disturbance in Prader–Willi syndrome. *American Journal of Medical Genetics*, **82**, 123–127.

Einfeld, S. L., Tonge, B. J. and Rees, V. W. (2001). Longitudinal course of behavioral and emotional problems in Williams syndrome. *American Journal of Mental Retardation*, **106**, 73–81.

Einfeld, S. L., Tonge, B. J., Turner, G. and Smith, E. (2004). Longitudinal course of behavioural and emotional problems in Prader–Willi, Fragile X, Williams and Down Syndromes. *Journal of Intellectual Disability Research*, **48**, 294.

Eldevik, S., Hastings, R. P., Hughes, J. C., Jahr, E., Eikeseth, S. and Cross, S. (2009). Meta-analysis of early intensive behavioral intervention for children with autism. *Journal of Clinical Child and Adolescent Psychology*, **38**, 439–450.

Emerson, E. (1990). Designing individualised community based placements as an alternative to institutions for people with a severe mental handicap and severe problem behaviour. In W. I. Fraser, ed. *Key Issues in Mental Retardation Research*. London: Routledge.

Emerson, E. (1995). *Challenging Behaviour: Analysis and Intervention in People with Intellectual Disabilities*. Cambridge: Cambridge University Press.

Emerson, E. (2001a). *Challenging Behaviour: Analysis and Intervention in People with Intellectual Disabilities*. Cambridge: Cambridge University Press.

Emerson, E. (2001b). Utilization of psychological services and psychological interventions by people with learning disabilities and challenging behaviour. *Clinical Psychology Review*, **8**, 25–29.

Emerson, E. (2002). The prevalence of use of reactive management strategies in community-based services in the UK. In D. Allen, ed. *Ethical Approaches to Physical Interventions: Responding to Challenging Behaviour in Persons with Intellectual Disabilities*. Kidderminster: BILD.

Emerson, E. (2003a). Prevalence of psychiatric disorders in children and adolescents with and without intellectual disability. *Journal of Intellectual Disability Research*, **47**, 51–58.

Emerson, E. (2003b). Mothers of children and adolescents with intellectual disability: social and economic situation, mental health status, and the self-assessed social and psychological impact of the child's difficulties. *Journal of Intellectual Disability Research*, **47**: Pt 4–5, 385–399.

Emerson, E. (2003c). Prevalence of psychiatric disorders in children and adolescents with and without intellectual disability. *Journal of Intellectual Disability Research*, **47**, 51–58.

Emerson, E. (2004). Poverty and children with intellectual disabilities in the world's richer countries. *Journal of Intellectual & Developmental Disability*, **29**, 319–337.

Emerson, E. (2006). The need for credible evidence: comments on 'on some recent claims for the efficacy of cognitive therapy for people with intellectual disabilities'. *Journal of Applied Research in Intellectual Disabilities*, **19**, 21–23.

Emerson, E. (2007). Poverty and people with intellectual disability. *Mental Retardation and Developmental Disabilities Research Reviews*, **13**, 107–113.

Emerson, E. (in press). Self-reported exposure to disablism is associated with poorer self-reported health and well-being among adults with intellectual disabilities in England: cross sectional survey. *Public Health*.

Emerson, E. and Howard, D. (1992). Schedule induced stereotypy. *Research in Developmental Disabilities*, **13**, 335–361.

Emerson, E. and Hatton, C. (1994). *Moving Out: The Impact of Relocation from Hospital to Community on the Quality of Life of People with Learning Disabilities*. London: HMSO.

Emerson, E. and Bromley, J. (1995). The form and function of challenging behaviours. *Journal of Intellectual Disability Research*, **39**, 388–398.

Emerson, E. and Hatton, C. (1996). Deinstitutionalization in the UK and Ireland: outcomes for service users. *Journal of Intellectual & Developmental Disability*: **21**, 17–37.

Emerson, E. and Hatton, C. (2007a). The contribution of socio-economic position to the health inequalities faced by children and adolescents with intellectual disabilities in Britain. *American Journal on Mental Retardation*, **112**, 140–150.

Emerson, E. and Hatton, C. (2007b). Poverty, socio-economic position, social capital and the health of children and adolescents with intellectual disabilities in Britain: a replication. *Journal of Intellectual Disability Research*, **51**, 866–874.

Emerson, E. and Hatton, C. (2007c). *The Mental Health of Children and Adolescents with Learning Disabilities in Britain*. London: Foundation for People with Learning Disabilities.

Emerson, E. and Hatton, C. (2007d). The mental health of children and adolescents with intellectual disabilities in Britain. *British Journal of Psychiatry*, **191**, 493–499.

Emerson, E. and Hatton, C. (2008a). Socioeconomic disadvantage, social participation and networks and the self-rated health of English men and women with mild and moderate intellectual disabilities: cross sectional survey. *European Journal of Public Health*, **18**, 31–37.

Emerson, E. and Hatton, C. (2008b). The self-reported well-being of women and men with intellectual disabilities in England. *American Journal on Mental Retardation*, **113**: 2, 143–155.

Emerson, E. and Robertson, J. (2008). Commissioning Person-centred, Cost-effective, Local Support for People with Learning Difficulties, London: SCIE.

Emerson, E. and Einfeld, S. (2010a). Emotional and behavioural difficulties in young children with and without developmental delay: A bi-national perspective. *Journal of Child Psychology and Psychiatry*, **51**, 583–593.

Emerson, E. and Hatton, C. (2010). Socio-economic position, poverty and family research. In L. M. Glidden and M. M. Seltzer, eds. *On Families: International Review of Research on Mental Retardation*. New York: Academic Press.

Emerson, E., Cummings, R., Barrett, S., Hughes, H., McCool, C. and Toogood, A. (1988). Challenging behaviour and community services: 2. Who are the people who challenge services? *Mental Handicap*, **16**, 16–19.

Emerson, E., McGill, P. and Mansell, J. (1994). *Severe Learning Disabilities and Challenging Behaviours: Designing High Quality Services*. London: Chapman & Hall.

Emerson, E., Thompson, S., Reeves, D., Henderson, D. and Robertson, J. (1995). Descriptive analysis of multiple response topographies of challenging behavior across two settings. *Research in Developmental Disabilities*, **16**, 301–329.

Emerson, E., Forrest, J., Cambridge, P. and Mansell, J. (1996a). Community support teams for people with learning disabilities and challenging behaviour: results of a National survey. *Journal of Mental Health*, **5**, 395–406.

Emerson, E., Reeves, D., Thompson, S., Henderson, D., Robertson, J. and Howard, D. (1996b). Time-based lag sequential analysis and the functional assessment of challenging behaviour. *Journal of Intellectual Disability Research*, **40**, 260–274.

Emerson, E., Thompson, S., Robertson, J. and Henderson, D. (1996c). Schedule-induced challenging behavior. *Journal of Developmental and Physical Disabilities*, **8**, 89–103.

Emerson, E., Hatton, C., Robertson, J., Henderson, D. and Cooper, J. (1999a). A descriptive analysis of the relationships between social context, engagement and stereotypy in residential services for people with severe and complex disabilities. *Journal of Applied Research in Intellectual Disabilities*, **12**, 11–29.

Emerson, E., Moss, S. and Kiernan, C. (1999b). The relationship between challenging behaviour and psychiatric disorder in people with severe developmental disabilities.

In N. Bouras, ed. *Psychiatric and Behavioural Disorders in Developmental Disabilities and Mental Retardation.* Cambridge: Cambridge University Press.

Emerson, E., Robertson, J., Hatton, C. *et al.* (1999c). Quality and Costs of Residential Supports for People With Learning Disabilities: Predicting Variation in Quality and Costs, Manchester: Hester Adrian Research Centre, University of Manchester.

Emerson, E., Robertson, J., Gregory, N. *et al.* (2000). The treatment and management of challenging behaviours in residential settings. *Journal of Applied Research in Intellectual Disabilities,* **13**, 197–215.

Emerson, E., Kiernan, C., Alborz, A. *et al.* (2001a). The prevalence of challenging behaviors: a total population study. *Research in Developmental Disabilities,* **22**: 1, 77–93.

Emerson, E., Kiernan, C., Alborz, A. *et al.* (2001b). Predicting the persistence of severe self-injurious behavior. *Research in Developmental Disabilities,* **22**: 1, 67–75.

Emerson, E., Robertson, J. and Wood, J. (2005). The mental health needs of children and adolescents with intellectual disabilities in an urban conurbation. *Journal of Intellectual Disability Research,* **49**, 16–24.

Emerson, E., Fujiura, G. T. and Hatton, C. (2007a). International perspectives. In S. L. Odom, R. H. Horner, M. Snell and J. Blacher, eds. *Handbook on Developmental Disabilities,* New York: Guilford Press.

Emerson, E., Robertson, J. and Wood, J. (2007b). The association between area-level indicators of social deprivation and the emotional and behavioural needs of black and South Asian children with intellectual disabilities in a deprived urban environment. *Journal of Applied Research in Intellectual Disabilities,* **20**, 420–429.

Emerson, E., McConkey, R., Walsh, P. and Felce, D. (2008). Intellectual disability in a global context. *Journal of Policy and Practice in Intellectual Disability,* **5**, 79–80.

Emerson, E., Graham, H., McCulloch, A., Blacher, J., Hatton, C. and Llewellyn, G. (2009). The social context of parenting three year old children with developmental delay in the UK. *Child: Care, Health & Development,* **35**: 1, 63–70.

Emerson, E., Einfeld, S. and Stancliffe, R. (2010). The mental health of young Australian children with intellectual disabilities or borderline intellectual functioning. *Social Psychiatry and Psychiatric Epidemiology,* **45**, 579–587.

Emerson, E., Einfeld, S. and Stancliffe, R. (in preparation). Persistence and emergence of conduct difficulties in children with borderline or intellectual disabilities.

Emerson, E., Einfeld, S. and Stancliffe, R. (2010). The mental health of young Australian children with intellectual disabilities or borderline intellectual functioning. *Social Psychiatry and Psychiatric Epidemiology,* **45**, 579–587.

English, C. L. and Anderson, C. M. (2006). Evaluation of the treatment utility of the analog functional analysis and the structured descriptive assessment. *Journal of Positive Behavior Interventions,* **8**, 212–229.

Esbensen, A. J. and Benson, B. A. (2006). A prospective analysis of life events, problem behaviours and depression in adults with intellectual disability. *Journal of Intellectual Disability Research,* **50**, 248–258.

Esbensen, A. J., Seltzer, M. M. and Krauss, M. W. (2008). Stability and change in health, functional abilities and behavior problems among adults with and without Down syndrome. *American Journal of Mental Retardation,* **113**, 263–277.

Espie, C. (1992). Optimal sleep-wake scheduling and profound mental handicap: potential benefits. *Mental Handicap*, **20**, 102–107.

Evans, G. W. and Kantrowitz, E. (2002). Socioeconomic status and health: the potential role of environmental risk exposure. *Annual Reviews of Public Health*, **23**, 303–331.

Evans, I. M. and Meyer, L. M. (1985). *An Educative Approach to Behavior Problems*. Baltimore: P.H. Brookes.

Eyman, R. K. and Call, T. (1977). Maladaptive behaviour and community placement of mentally retarded persons. *American Journal of Mental Deficiency*, **82**, 137–144.

Eyman, R. K., Borthwick, S. A. and Miller, C. (1981). Trends in maladaptive behavior of mentally retarded persons placed in community and institutional settings. *American Journal of Mental Deficiency* **85**, 473–477.

Fabian Commission on Life Chances and Child Poverty (2006). *Narrowing the Gap: The Final Report of the Fabian Commission on Life Chances and Child Poverty*. London: Fabian Society.

Favell, J. E., McGimsey, J. F. and Schell, R. M. (1982). Treatment of self injury by providing alternate sensory activities. *Analysis and Intervention in Developmental Disabilities*, **2**, 83–104.

Felce, D., Lowe, K., Perry, J. *et al.* (1998). Service support to people in Wales with severe intellectual disability and the most severe challenging behaviours: processes, outcomes and costs. *Journal of Intellectual Disability Research*, **42**, 390–408.

Feldman, M. A. and Griffiths, D. (1997). Comprehensive assessment of severe behavior problems. In N. N. Singh, ed. *Prevention and Treatment of Severe Behavior Problems: Models and Methods in Developmental Disabilities*. Pacific Grove: Brooks/Cole.

Feldman, M. A., Atkinson, L., Foti-Gervais, L. and Condillac, R. (2004). Formal versus informal interventions for challenging behaviours in persons with intellectual disabilities. *Journal of Intellectual Disability Research*, **48**, 60–68.

Ferro, J., Foster-Johnson, L. and Dunlap, G. (1996). Relation between curricular activities and problem behaviors of students with mental retardation. *American Journal of Mental Retardation*, **101**, 184–194.

Fisch, G. S., Simensen, R. J. and Schroer, R. J. (2002). Longitudinal changes in cognitive and adaptive behavior scores in children and adolescents with the Fragile X mutation or autism. *Journal of Autism and Developmental Disorders*, **32**, 107–114.

Fisher, W., Piazza, C., Cataldo, M., Harrell, R., Jefferson, G. and Conner, R. (1993). Functional communication training with and without extinction and punishment. *Journal of Applied Behavior Analysis*, **26**, 23–36.

Fisher, W. W. and Mazur, J. E. (1997). Basic and applied research on choice responding. *Journal of Applied Behavior Analysis*, **30**, 387–410.

Floyd, F. J. and Saitzyk, A. R. (1992). Social class and parenting children with mild and moderate mental retardation. *Journal of Pediatric Psychology*, **17**, 607–631.

Forehand, R. and Baumeister, A. A. (1970). The effect of auditory and visual stimulation on stereotyped rocking behavior and general activity of severe retardates. *Journal of Clinical Psychology*, **26**, 426–429.

Foster-Johnson, L., Ferro, J. and Dunlap, G. (1994). Preferred curricular activities and reduced problem behaviors in students with intellectual disabilities. *Journal of Applied Behavior Analysis*, **27**, 493–504.

Fox, P. and Emerson, E. (2001). Socially valid outcomes of intervention for people with mental retardation and challenging behavior: a preliminary descriptive analysis of the views of different stakeholders. *Journal of Positive Behavior Interventions*, 3, 183–189.

Fox, P. and Emerson, E. (2002). *Positive Outcomes*. Brighton: Pavilion Press.

Fox, P. and Emerson, E. (in press). *Positive Outcomes*. Brighton: Pavilion Press.

Foxx, R. M. (1990). Harry: a ten year follow up of the successful treatment of a self injurious man. *Research in Developmental Disabilities*, 11, 67–76.

Freeman, K., Walker, M. and Kaufman, J. (2007). Psychometric properties of the Questions About Behavioral Functions Scale. *American Journal on Mental Retardation*, 112, 122–129.

Friedli, L. (2009). *Mental Health, Resilience and Inequalities*. Copenhagen: World Health Organization, Europe.

Friman, P. C. and Hawkins, R. O. (2006). Contribution of establishing operations to antecedent intervention: clinical implications and motivating events. In J. K. Luiselli, ed. *Antecedent Assessment and Intervention*. Baltimore: Paul H Brookes.

Fujiura, G. T. (1998). Demography of family households. *American Journal on Mental Retardation*, 103, 225–235.

G. Allen Roeher Institute (1988). *The Language of Pain: Perspectives on Behavior Management*. Downsview, Ont: G. Allen Roeher Institute.

Gardner, W. I. and Whalen, J. P. (1996). A multimodal behavior analytic model for evaluating the effects of medical problems on nonspecific behavioral symptoms in persons with developmental disabilities. *Behavioral Interventions*, 11, 147–161.

Gardner, W. I., Karan, O. C. and Cole, C. L. (1984). Assessment of setting events influencing functional capacities of mentally retarded adults with behavior difficulties. In A. S. Halpern and M. J. Fuhrer, eds. *Functional Assessment in Rehabilitation*. Baltimore: Brookes.

Gardner, W. I., Cole, C. L., Davidson, D. P. and Karan, O. C. (1986). Reducing aggression in individuals with developmental disabilities: an expanded stimulus control, assessment, and intervention model. *Education and Training of the Mentally Retarded*, 21, 3–12.

Gary, L. A., Tallon, R. J. and Stangl, J. M. (1980). Environmental influences on self-stimulatory behavior. *American Journal of Mental Deficiency*, 85, 171–175.

Gaskin, C. J., Elsom, S. J. and Happell, B. (2007). Interventions for reducing seclusion in psychiatric facilities. *British Journal of Psychiatry*, 191, 298–303.

Gedye, A. (1989a). Extreme self injury attributed to frontal lobe seizures. *American Journal on Mental Retardation*, 94, 20–26.

Gedye, A. (1989b). Episodic rage and aggression attributed to frontal lobe seizures. *Journal of Mental Deficiency Research*, 33, 369–379.

Ghate, D. and Hazel, N. (2002). *Parenting in Poor Environments: Stress, Support and Coping*. London: Jessica Kingsley.

Glaser, D. (2008). Child sexual abuse. In M. Rutter, D. Bihop, D. Pine, *et al.*, eds. *Rutter's Child and Adolescent Psychiatry*. Oxford: Blackwell.

Glaser, E. M., Abelson, H. H. and Garrison, K. N. (1983). *Putting Knowledge to Use: Facilitating the Diffusion of Knowledge and the Implementation of Planned Change*. San Francisco: Jossey-Bass.

Glasgow, R. E., Vogt, T. M. and Boles, S. M. (1999). Evaluating the public health impact of health promotion interventions: the RE-AIM framework. *American Journal of Public Health*, **89**, 1322–1327.

Goldiamond, I. (1974). Toward a constructional approach to social problems: ethical and constitutional issues raised by applied behavior analysis. *Behaviorism*, **2**, 1–84.

Golding, L., Emerson, E. and Thornton, A. (2005). An evaluation of specialized community-based residential supports for people with challenging behavior. *Journal of Intellectual Disabilities*, **92**, 145–154.

Goldstein, S. and Brooks, R. B. (2006). *Handbook of Resilience in Children*. New York: Springer.

Goodman, R. (1999). The extended version of the Strengths and Difficulties Questionnaire as a guide to child psychiatric caseness and consequent burden. *Journal of Child Psychology and Psychiatry*, **40**, 791–801.

Graham, H. (2007). *Unequal Lives: Health and Socioeconomic Inequalities*. Maidenhead: Open University Press.

Grant, K. E., Compas, B. E., Thurm, A. E. *et al.* (2006). Stressors and child and adolescent psychopathology: evidence of moderating and mediating effects. *Clinical Psychology Review*, **26**, 257–283.

Green, C. W., Gardner, S. M., Canipe, V. S. and Reid, D. H. (1994). Analyzing alertness among people with profound multiple disabilities: Implications for provision of training. *Journal of Applied Behavior Analysis*, **27**, 519–531.

Green, L. (2006). Public health asks of systems science: to advance our evidence-based practice, can you help us get more practice-based evidence? *American Journal of Public Health*, **96**, 406–409.

Green, V. A., O'Reilly, M., Itchon, J. and Sigafoos, J. (2005). Persistence of early emerging aberrant behavior in children with developmental disabilities. *Research in Developmental Disabilities*, **26**, 47–55.

Groark, C. J. and McCall, R. B. (2008). Community-based interventions and services. In M. Rutter, D. Bishop, D. Pine *et al.* eds. *Rutter's Child and Adolescent Psychiatry*. London: Blackwell.

Guess, D. and Carr, E. G. (1991). Emergence and maintenance of stereotypy and self injury. *American Journal on Mental Retardation*, **96**, 299–319.

Guess, D., Helmstetter, H., Turnbull, H. R. and Knowlton, S. (1987). *Use of aversive procedures with persons who are disabled: an historical review and critical analysis.* Seattle, WA: The Association for Persons with Severe Handicaps.

Guess, D., Siegel-Causey, E., Roberts, S., Rues, J., Thompson, B. and Siegel-Causey, D. (1990). Assessment and analysis of behavior state and related variables among students with profoundly handicapping conditions. *Journal of the Association for Persons with Severe Handicaps*, **15**, 211–230.

Gunn, P., Berry, P. and Andrews, R. J. (1981). The temperament of Down's syndrome infants: a research note. *Journal of Child Psychology and Psychiatry*, **22**, 189–194.

Guralnick, M. J. (1997). *The Effectiveness of Early Intervention*. Baltimore: Brookes/Cole.

Guralnick, M. J. (2005). Early intervention for children with intellectual disabilities: current knowledge and future prospect. *Journal of Applied Research in Intellectual Disabilities*, **18**, 313–323.

Hagerman, R. and Hagerman, P. (2002). Fragile X syndrome. In P. Howlin and O. Udwin, eds. *Outcomes in Neurodevelopmental and Genetic Disorders*. Cambridge: Cambridge University Press.

Hagopian, L. P., Fisher, W. W. and Legacy, S. M. (1994). Schedule effects of noncontingent reinforcement on attention-maintained destructive behavior in identical quadruplets. *Journal of Applied Behavior Analysis*, **27**, 317–325.

Hall, S. and Oliver, C. (1992). Differential effects of severe self injurious behaviour on the behaviour of others. *Behavioural Psychotherapy*, **20**, 355–365.

Hall, S. and Oliver, C. (2000). An alternative approach to the sequential analysis of behavioral interactions. In T. Thompson, D. Felce and F. Symons, eds. *Computer Assisted Behavioral Observation Methods for Developmental Disabilities*. Baltimore: Paul H Brookes.

Hall, S. S., Arron, K., Sloneem, J. and Oliver, C. (2008). Health and sleep problems in Cornelia de Lange Syndrome: a case control study. *Journal of Intellectual Disability Research*, **52**, 458–468.

Hamilton, D., Sutherland, G. and Iacono, T. (2005). Further examination of relationships between life events and psychiatric symptoms in adults with intellectual disability. *Journal of Intellectual Disability Research*, **49**, 839–844.

Hanley, G. P., Piazza, C. C., Fisher, W. W., Contrucci, S. A. and Maglieri, K. A. (1997). Evaluation of client preference for function-based treatment packages. *Journal of Applied Behavior Analysis*, **30**, 459–473.

Hanley, G. P., Iwata, B. A. and McCord, B. E. (2003). Functional analysis of problem behavior: a review. *Journal of Applied Behavior Analysis*, **36**, 147–185.

Harchik, A. E. and Putzier, V. S. (1990). The use of high-probability requests to increase compliance with instructions to take medication. *Journal of the Association for Persons with Severe Handicaps*, **15**, 40–43.

Hardan, A. and Sahl, R. (1997). Psychopathology in children and adolescents with developmental disorders. *Research in Developmental Disabilities*, **18**, 369–382.

Harris, J., Cornick, M., Jefferson, A. and Mills, R. (2008). *Physical Interventions. A Policy Framework*. Kidderminster: BILD Publications.

Harris, J. C. (2005). *Intellectual Disability: Understanding Its Development, Causes, Evaluation, and Treatment*. Oxford: Oxford University Press.

Harris, P. (1993). The nature and extent of aggressive behaviour among people with learning difficulties (mental handicap) in a single health district. *Journal of Intellectual Disability Research*, **37**, 221–242.

Harris, P. and Russell, O. (1998). The prevalence of aggressive behaviour among people with learning difficulties (mental handicap) in a single health district. Bristol: Norah Fry Research Centre: University of Bristol.

Harris, S. L., Alessandri, M. I. and Gill, M. J. (1991). Training parents of developmentally disabled children. In J. L. Matson and J. A. Mulick, eds. *Handbook of Mental Retardation*. New York: Pergamon.

Harvey, S. T., Boer, D., Meyer, L. H. and Evans, I. M. (2009). Updating a meta-analysis of intervention research with challenging behaviour: Treatment validity and standards of practice. *Journal of Intellectual & Developmental Disability*, **34**, 67–80.

Haskett, M. E., Nears, K., Ward, C. A. and McPherson, A. V. (2006). Diversity in adjustment of maltreated children: factors associated with resilient functioning. *Clinical Psychology Review*, **26**, 796–812.

Hassiotis, A., Robotham, D., Canagasabey, A. *et al.* (2009). Randomized, single-blind, controlled trial of a specialist behavior therapy team for challenging behavior in adults with intellectual disabilities. *American Journal of Psychiatry*, **166**, 1278–1285.

Hastings, R. P. (2002). Parental stress and behaviour problems in children with developmental disability. *Journal of Intellectual and Developmental Disability*, **27**, 149–160.

Hastings, R. P. and Remington, B. (1994). Rules of engagement: Toward an analysis of staff responses to challenging behaviour. *Research in Developmental Disabilities*, **15**, 279–298.

Hastings, R. P., Hatton, C., Taylor, J. L. and Maddison, C. (2004). Life events and psychiatric symptoms in adults with intellectual disabilities. *Journal of Intellectual Disability Research* **48**, 42–46.

Hatton, C. (2004). Choice. In E. Emerson, C. Hatton, T. Thompson and T. Parmenter, eds. *International Handbook of Applied Research in Intellectual Disabilities*. Chichester: Wiley.

Hatton, C. and Emerson, E. (2004). The relationship between life events and psychopathology amongst children with intellectual disabilities. *Journal of Applied Research in Intellectual Disabilities*, **17**, 109–118.

Hatton, C., Emerson, E., Kirby, S. *et al.* (2010). Majority and minority ethnic family carers of adults with intellectual disabilities: perceptions of challenging behaviour and family impact. *Journal of Applied Research in Intellectual Disabilities*, **23**, 63–74.

Hawkins, S., Allen, D. and Jenkins, R. (2005). The use of physical interventions with people with intellectual disabilities and challenging behaviour – the experience of service users and staff members. *Journal of Applied Research in Intellectual Disabilities*, **18**, 19–34.

Hayes, S. C. (1989). *Rule Governed Behavior: Cognition, Contingencies and Instructional Control.* New York: Plenum.

Haynes, B. (1999). Can it work? Does it work? Is it worth it? *British Medical Journal*, **319**, 676–677.

Heber, R. (1970). *Epidemiology of Mental Retardation.* Springfield, Ill: Thomas.

Heidorn, S. D. and Jensen, C. C. (1984). Generalization and maintenance of the reduction of self-injurious behavior maintained by two types of reinforcement. *Behaviour Research and Therapy*, **22**, 581–586.

Heikura, U., Taanila, A. and Hartikainen, A.-L. (2008). Variations in prenatal sociodemographic factors associated with intellectual disability: a study of the 20-Year interval between two birth cohorts in Northern Finland. *American Journal of Epidemiology*, **167**, 169–177.

Hemmings, C. (2007). The relationship between challenging behaviours and psychiatric disorders in people with severe disabilities. In N. Bouras and G. Holt, eds. *Psychiatric and Behavioural Disorders in Intellectual and Developmental Disabilities*. Cambridge: Cambridge University Press.

Hill, B. K. and Bruininks, R. H. (1984). Maladaptive behavior of mentally retarded individuals in residential facilities. *American Journal of Mental Deficiency*, **88**, 380–387.

Hogg, J. and Langa, A. (2005). *Assessing Adults with Intellectual Disabilities.* Oxford: Blackwell.

Holden, B. and Gitlesen, J. P. (2004). Psychotropic medication in adults with mental retardation: prevalence, and prescription practices. *Research in Developmental Disabilities*, **25**, 509–521.

Holden, B. and Gitlesen, J. P. (2006). A total population study of challenging behaviour in the county of Hedmark, Norway: prevalence, and risk markers. *Research in Developmental Disabilities*, **27**, 456–465.

Holland, A., Whittington, J. and Hinton, E. (2003). The paradox of Prader–Willi syndrome: a genetic model of starvation. *Lancet*, **362**, 989–991.

Horner, R. D. (1980). The effects of an environmental 'enrichment' program on the behavior of institutionalized profoundly retarded children. *Journal of Applied Behavior Analysis*, **13**, 473–491.

Horner, R. H., Sprague, J. R., O'Brien, M. and Heathfield, L. T. (1990). The role of response efficiency in the reduction of problem behaviors through functional equivalence training: a case study. *Journal of the Association for Persons with Severe Handicaps*, **15**, 91–97.

Horner, R. H., Day, H. M., Sprague, J. R., O'Brien, M. and Heathfield, L. T. (1991). Interspersed requests: a nonaversive procedure for reducing aggression and self-injury during instruction. *Journal of Applied Behavior Analysis*, **24**, 265–278.

Horner, R. H., Day, H. M. and Day, J. R. (1997). Using neutralizing routines to reduce problem behaviors. *Journal of Applied Behavior Analysis*, **30**, 601–614.

Horner, R. H., Sugai, G., Smolkowski, K. *et al.* (2009). A randomized wait-list controlled effectiveness trial assessing school-wide positive behavior support in elementary classrooms. *Journal of Positive Behavior Interventions*, **11**, 133–144.

Horsler, K. and Oliver, C. (2006). Environmental influences on the behavioural phenotype of Angelman syndrome. *American Journal on Mental Retardation*, **11**, 311–321.

Hosman, C. M. H., Jane-Llopis, E. and Saxena, S. (2005). *Prevention of Mental Disorders: Effective Interventions and Policy Options*. Oxford: Oxford University Press.

Huckshorn, K. A. (2005). *Six Core Strategies to Reduce the Use of Seclusion and Restraint Planning Tool*. Alexandria, VA: National Technical Assistance Centre.

Hudson, A., Wilken, P. and Jauering, R. (1995). Regionally based teams for the treatment of challenging behaviour: a three year outcome study. *Behavioural Change*, **12**, 209–215.

Hulbert-Williams, L. and Hastings, R. P. (2008). Life events as a risk factor for psychological problems in individuals with intellectual disabilities: a critical review. *Journal of Intellectual Disability Research*, **52**, 883–895.

Hutchinson, R. R. (1977). By products of aversive control. In W. K. Honig and J. E. R. Staddon, eds. *Handbook of Operant Behavior*. Englewood Cliffs, NJ: Prentice Hall.

Institute of Medicine (2001). *Neurological, Psychiatric, and Developmental Disorders: Meeting the Challenge in the Developing World*. Washington, DC: National Academy Press.

Irwin, L. G., Siddiqi, A. and Hertzman, C. (2007). *Early Child Development : A Powerful Equalizer*. Geneva: World Health Organisation.

Iwata, B. A. (1988). The development and adoption of controversial default technologies. *The Behavior Analyst*, **11**, 149–157.

Iwata, B. A., Dorsey, M. F., Slifer, K. J., Bauman, K E. and Richman, G. S. (1982). Toward a functional analysis of self injury. *Analysis and Intervention in Developmental Disabilities*, **2**, 3–20.

Iwata, B. A., Pace, G. M., Cowdery, G. E. and Miltenberger, R. G. (1994a). What makes extinction work: an analysis of procedural form and function. *Journal of Applied Behavior Analysis*, **27**, 131–144.

Iwata, B. A., Pace, G. M., Dorsey, M. F. *et al.* (1994b). The functions of self injurious behavior: an experimental epidemiological study. *Journal of Applied Behavior Analysis*, **27**, 215–240.

Iwata, B. A., Smith, R. G. and Michael, J. (2000). Current research on the influence of establishing operations on behavior in applied settings. *Journal of Applied Behavior Analysis*, **33**, 411–418.

Jacobsen, J. W., Silver, E. J. and Schwartz, A. A. (1984). Service provision in New York's group homes. *Mental Retardation*, **22**, 231–239.

Jarjoura, G. R., Triplett, R. A. and Brinker, G. P. (2002). Growing up poor: Examining the link between persistent childhood poverty and delinquency. *Journal of Quantitative Criminology*, **18**, 159–187.

Jenkins, J. (2008). Psychosocial adversity and resilience. In M. Rutter, D. Bishop, D. Pine *et al.*, eds. *Rutter's Child and Adolescent Psychiatry*. 5th edn. Oxford: Blackwell.

Jenkins, R., Rose, J. and Lovell, C. (1997). Psychological well-being of staff working with people who have challenging behaviour. *Journal of Intellectual Disability Research*, **41**, 502–511.

Jensen, C. C. and Heidorn, S. D. (1993). Ten year follow up of a successful treatment of self injurious behavior. *Behavioral Residential Treatment*, **8**, 263–280.

Jones, D. P. H. (2008). Child maltreatment. In M. Rutter, D. Bishop, D. Pine *et al.*, eds. *Rutter's Child and Adolescent Psychiatry*. Oxford: Blackwell.

Jones, E., Felce, D., Lowe, K. *et al.* (2001). Evaluation of the dissemination of active support training in staffed community residences. *American Journal on Mental Retardation*, **106**, 344–358.

Jones, E., Allen, D., Moore, K., Phillips, B. and Lowe, K. (2007). Restraint and self-injury in people with intellectual disabilities. *Journal of Intellectual Disabilities*, **2**, 1–13.

Jones, P. and Kroese, B. S. (2006). Service users' views of physical restraint procedures in secure settings for people with learning disabilities. *British Journal of Learning Disabilities*, **35**, 50–54.

Kahng, S., Iwata, B. A., Fischer, S. M. *et al.* (1998). Temporal distributions of problem behavior based on scatter plot analysis. *Journal of Applied Behavior Analysis*, **31**, 593–604.

Kalachnik, J. E., Hanzel, T. E., Harder, S. R., Bauernfeind, J. D. and Engstrom, E. A. (1995). Antiepileptic drug behavioral side effects in individuals with mental retardation and the use of behavioral measurement techniques. *Mental Retardation*, **33**, 374–382.

Kalachnik, J. E., Leventhal, B. L., James, D. J. *et al.* (1998). Guidelines for the use of psychotropic medication. In S. Reiss and M. G. Aman, eds. *Psychotropic Medication and Developmental Disabilities: The International Consensus Handbook*. Ohio: Nisonger Center, Ohio State University.

Kantor, J. R. (1959). *Interbehavioral Psychology*. Chicago: Principa Press.

Kawachi, I. and Berkman, L. F. (2003). *Neighborhoods and Health*. Oxford: Oxford University Press.

Kazdin, A. E. and Matson, J. L. (1981). Social validation in mental retardation. *Applied Research in Mental Retardation*, 2, 39–53.

Kearney, C. A. (1994). Interrater reliability of the Motivation Assessment Scale: another, closer look. *Journal of the Association for Persons with Severe Handicaps*, 19, 139–142.

Kennedy, C. H. (1994a). Manipulating antecedent conditions to alter the stimulus control of problem behavior. *Journal of Applied Behavior Analysis*, 27, 161–170.

Kennedy, C. H. (1994b). Automatic reinforcement: oxymoron or hypothetical construct? *Journal of Behavioral Education*, 4, 387–395.

Kennedy, C. H. (2002). Evolution of stereotypy into self-injury. In S. R. Schroeder, M. L. Oster-Granite and T. Thompson, eds. *Self-Injurious Behavior: Gene–Brain–Behavior Relationships*. Washington, DC: American Psychological Association.

Kennedy, C. H. and Itkonen, T. (1993). Effects of setting events on the problem behavior of students with severe disabilities. *Journal of Applied Behavior Analysis*, 26, 321–327.

Kennedy, C. H. and Meyer, K. A. (1996). Sleep deprivation, allergy symptoms, and negatively reinforced problem behavior. *Journal of Applied Behavior Analysis*, 29, 133–135.

Kennedy, C. H. and Meyer, K. A. (1998). Establishing operations and the motivation of challenging behavior. In J. K. Luiselli and M. J. Cameron, eds. *Antecedent Control: Innovative Approaches to Behavioral Support*. Baltimore: Paul H Brookes.

Kennedy, C. H. and Becker, A. (2006). Health conditions in antecedent assessment and intervention of problem behavior. In J. Luiselli, ed. *Antecedent Assessment and Intervention*. Baltimore: Brookes.

Kern, L., Koegel, R. L., Dyer, K., Blew, P. A. and Fenton, L. R. (1982). The effects of physical exercise on self-stimulation and appropriate responding in autistic children. *Journal of Autism and Developmental Disorders*, 12, 399–419.

Kern, L., Koegel, R. L. and Dunlap, G. (1984). The influence of vigorous versus mild exercise on autistic stereotyped behaviors. *Journal of Autism and Developmental Disorders*, 14, 57–67.

Kern, L., Sokol, N. G. and Dunlap, G. (2006). Assessment of antecedent influences on challenging behavior. In J. Luiselli, ed. *Antecedent Assessment and Intervention*. Baltimore: Brookes.

Kiernan, C. and Qureshi, H. (1993). Challenging behaviour. In C. Kiernan, ed. *Research to Practice? Implications of Research on the Challenging Behaviour of People with Learning Disabilities*. Kidderminster: British Institute of Learning Disabilities.

Kiernan, C. and Kiernan, D. (1994). Challenging behaviour in schools for pupils with severe learning difficulties. *Mental Handicap Research*, 7, 117–201.

Kiernan, C. and Alborz, A. (1996). Persistence and change in challenging and problem behaviours of young adults with learning disability of young adults living in the family home. *Journal of Applied Research in Intellectual Disability*, 9, 181–193.

Kiernan, C., Reeves, D. and Alborz, A. (1995). The use of anti-psychotic drugs with adults with learning disabilities and challenging behaviour. *Journal of Intellectual Disability Research*, 39, 263–274.

Kiernan, C., Reeves, D., Hatton, C. *et al.* (1997). The HARC Challenging Behaviour Project. Report 1: Persistence and change in the challenging behaviour of people with learning disability, Manchester: Hester Adrian Research Centre, University of Manchester.

Kim, S., Larson, S. A. and Lakin, K. C. (2001). Behavioural outcomes of deinstitutionalisation for people with intellectual disability: a review of studies conducted between 1980 and 1999. *Journal of Intellectual & Developmental Disability*, **26**, 35–50.

Knobbe, C., Carey, S., Rhodes, L. and Horner, R. (1995). Benefit–cost analysis of community residential versus institutional services for adults with severe mental retardation and challenging behaviors. *American Journal on Mental Retardation*, **99**, 533–541.

Koegel, L. K., Koegel, R. L. and Dunlap, G. (1996). *Positive Behavioral Support: Including People With Difficult Behavior in the Community*. Baltimore: Brookes.

Koegel, R. L. and Koegel, L. K. (1988). Generalized responsivity and pivotal behaviors. In R. H. Horner, G. Dunlap and R. L. Koegel, eds. *Generalization and Maintenance: Life-Style Changes in Applied Settings*. Baltimore: Paul H Brookes.

Koegel, R. L. and Koegel, L. K. (1990). Extended reductions in stereotypic behavior of students with autism through a self- management treatment package. *Journal of Applied Behavior Analysis*, **23**, 119–127.

Konarski, E. A., Sutton, K. and Huffman, A. (1997). Personal characteristics associated with episodes of injury in a residential facility. *American Journal of Mental Retardation*, **102**, 37–44.

Koskentausta, T., Iivanainen, M. and Almqvist, F. (2006). Risk factors for psychiatric disturbance in children with intellectual disability. *Journal of Intellectual Disability Research*, **51**, 43–53.

Kozma, A., Mansell, J. and Beadle-Brown, J. (2009). Outcomes in different residential settings for people with intellectual disability: a systematic review. *American Journal on Intellectual and Developmental Disabilities*, **114**, 193–222.

Krantz, P. and Risley, T. R. (1977). Behavioral ecology in the classroom. In S. G. O' Leary and K. D. O' Leary, eds. *Classroom Management: The Successful Use of Behavior Modification*. New York: Pergamon.

Kroese, B. S., Dagnan, D. and Loumidis, K. (1997). *Cognitive Behaviour Therapy for People with Intellectual Disabilities*. London: Routledge.

Kuhn, D. E., Hardesty, S. L. and Luczynski, K. (2009). Further evaluation of antecedent social events during functional analysis. *Journal of Applied Behavior Analysis*, **42**, 349–353.

Kurtz, P. F., Chin, M. D., Huete, J. M. *et al.* (2003). Functional analysis and treatment of self-injurious behavior in young children: a summary of 30 cases. *Journal of Applied Behavior Analysis*, **36**, 205–219.

Lancaster, G. A., Whittington, R., Lane, S., Riley, D. and Meehan, C. (2008). Does the position of restraint of disturbed psychiatric patients have any association with staff and patient injuries? *Journal of Psychiatric and Mental Health Nursing*, **15**, 306–312.

Lancioni, G., O'Reilly, M. F., Campodonico, F. and Mantini, M. (1998). Task variation versus task repetition for people with profound developmental disabilities: an assessment of preferences. *Research in Developmental Disabilities*, **19**, 189–199.

Lancioni, G. E. and O'Reilly, M. F. (1998). A review of research on physical exercise with people with severe and profound developmental disabilities. *Research in Developmental Disabilities*, **19**, 477–492.

Lancioni, G. E., O'Reilly, M. F. and Emerson, E. (1996). A review of choice research with people with severe and profound developmental disabilities. *Research in Developmental Disabilities*, **17**, 391–411.

Lancioni, G. E., O'Reilly, M. F. and Basili, G. (1999). Review of strategies for treating sleep problems in persons with severe or profound mental retardation or multiple handicaps. *American Journal of Mental Retardation*, **104**, 170–186.

Lang, R., O'Reilly, M., Machalicek, W., Lancioni, G., Rispoli, M. and Chan, J. M. (2008). A preliminary comparison of functional analysis results when conducted in contrived versus natural settings. *Journal of Applied Behavior Analysis*, **41**, 441–445.

Lang, R., O'Reilly, M., Lancioni, G. *et al.* (2009a). Discrepancy in functional analysis results across two settings: Implications for intervention design. *Journal of Applied Behavior Analysis*, **42**, 393–397.

Lang, R., Rispoli, M., Machalicek, W. *et al.* (2009b). Treatment of elopement in individuals with developmental disabilities: a systematic review. *Research in Developmental Disabilities*, **30**, 670–681.

Langee, H. R. (1990). Retrospective study of lithium use for institutionalized mentally retarded individuals with behaviour disorders. *American Journal on Mental Retardation*, **94**, 448–452.

Langthorne, P. and McGill, P. (2008). Functional analysis of the early development of self-injurious behaviour: incorporating gene–environment interactions. *American Journal of Mental Retardation*, **113**, 403–417.

Laraway, S., Snycerski, S., Michael, J. and Poling, A. (2003). Motivating operations and terms to describe them: some further refinements. *Journal of Applied Behavior Analysis*, **36**, 407–414.

LaVigna, G. W. and Willis, T. J. (1994). *Positive Strategies for Severe and Challenging Behaviour*. Los Angeles: Institute for Applied Behaviour Analysis.

LaVigna, G. W. and Willis, T. J. (2002). Counter-intuitive strategies for crisis management within a non-aversive framework. In D. Allen, ed. *Ethical Approaches to Physical Intervention. Responding to Challenging Behaviour in People with Intellectual Disabilities*. Kidderminster: BILD Publications.

LaVigna, G. W., Willis, T. J. and Donnellan, A. M. (1989). The role of positive programming in behavioural treatment. In E. Cipani, ed. *The Treatment of Severe Behaviour Disorders*. Washington: American Association on Mental Retardation.

Leggett, J. and Silvester, J. (2003). Care staff attributions for violent incidents involving male and female patients: a field study. *British Journal of Clinical Psychology*, **42**, 393–406.

Leonard, H. and Wen, X. (2002). The epidemiology of mental retardation: challenges and opportunities in the new millennium. *Mental Retardation and Developmental Disabilities Research Reviews*, **8**, 117–134.

Lerman, D. C. and Iwata, B. A. (1995). Prevalence of the extinction burst and its attenuation during treatment. *Journal of Applied Behavior Analysis*, **28**, 93–94.

Lerman, D. C. and Iwata, B. A. (1996). Developing a technology for the use of operant extinction in clinical settings: an examination of basic and applied research. *Journal of Applied Behavior Analysis*, **29**, 345–382.

Lerman, D. C., Iwata, B. A., Zarcone, J. R. and Ringdahl, J. (1994). Assessment of stereo-typic and self-injurious behavior as adjunctive responses. *Journal of Applied Behavior Analysis*, 27, 715–728.

Leudar, I., Fraser, W. I. and Jeeves, M. A. (1984). Behaviour disturbance and mental handicap: typology and longitudinal trends. *Psychological Medicine*, 14, 923–935.

Lewis, J. N., Tonge, B. J., Mowat, D. R., Einfeld, S. L., Siddons, H. M. and Rees, V. W. (2000). Epilepsy and associated psychopathology in young people with intellectual disability. *Journal of Paediatrics and Child Health*, 36, 172–175.

Lewis, M. H., Bodfish, J. W., Powell, S. B. and Golden, R. N. (1995). Clomipramine treatment for stereotype and related repetitive movement disorders associated with mental retardation. *American Journal of Mental Retardation*, 100, 299–312.

Lindauer, S. E., DeLeon, I. G. and Fisher, W. W. (1999). Decreasing signs of negative affect and correlated self-injury in an individual with mental retardation and mood disturbances. *Journal of Applied Behavior Analysis*, 32, 103–106.

Linscheid, T. R. (1992). Aversive stimulation. In J. K. Luiselli, J. L. Matson and N. N. Singh, eds. *Self-Injurious Behavior: Analysis, Assessment and Treatment*. New York: Springer-Verlag.

Linver, M. R., Brooks-Gunn, J. and Kohen, D. E. (2002). Family processes as pathways from income to young children's development. *Developmental Psychology*, 38, 719–743.

Lister, R. (2004). *Poverty*, Cambridge: Polity Press.

Llewellyn, G., McConnell, D., Thompson, K. and Whybrow, S. (2005). Out-of-home placement of school-age children with disabilities. *Journal of Applied Research in Intellectual Disability*, 18, 1–6.

Loeber, R. and Hay, D. F. (1997). Key issues in the development of aggression and violence from childhood to early adulthood. *Annual Review of Psychology*, 48, 371–410.

Loesch, D. Z., Huggins, R. M. and Hagerman, R. J. (2004). Phenotypic variation and FMRP levels in Fragile X. *Mental Retardation and Developmental Disabilities Research Reviews*, 10, 31–41.

Lovaas, O. I. (1982). Comments on self destructive behaviors. *Analysis and Intervention in Developmental Disabilities*, 2, 115–124.

Lovaas, O. I. and Simmons, J. Q. (1969). Manipulation of self destructive behavior in three retarded children. *Journal of Applied Behavior Analysis*, 2, 143–157.

Lovaas, O. I., Freitag, G., Gold, V. J. and Kassorla, I. C. (1965). Experimental studies in childhood schitzophrenia: analysis of self destructive behavior. *Journal of Experimental Child Psychology*, 2, 67–84.

Lovaas, O. I., Newsom, C. and Hickman, C. (1987). Self stimulatory behavior and perceptual reinforcement. *Journal of Applied Behavior Analysis*, 20, 45–68.

Lowe, C. F. (1979). Determinants of human operant behavior. In M. D. Zeilor and P. Harjem, eds. *Reinforcement and the Organization of Behavior*. Chichester: Wiley.

Lowe, K. and Felce, D. (1995a). The definition of challenging behaviour in practice. *British Journal of Learning Disabilities*, 23, 118–123.

Lowe, K. and Felce, D. (1995b). How do carers assess the severity of challenging behaviour? A total population study. *Journal of Intellectual Disability Research*, 39, 117–128.

Lowe, K., Felce, D. and Blackman, D. (1996). Challenging behaviour: the effectiveness of specialist support teams. *Journal of Intellectual Disability Research*, **40**: 336–347.

Lowe, K., Allen, D., Brophy, S. and Moore, K. (2005). The management and treatment of challenging behaviours. *Tizard Learning Disability Review*, **10**, 34–37.

Lowe, K., Allen, D., Jones, E., Brophy, S., Moore, K. and James, W. (2007). Challenging behaviours: prevalence and topographies. *Journal of Intellectual Disability Research*, **51**, 625–636.

Lowry, M. A. and Sovner, R. (1992). Severe behavior problems associated rapid cycling bipolar disorder in two adults with profound mental retardation. *Journal of Intellectual Disability Research*, **36**, 269–281.

Luckasson, R., Borthwick Duffy, S. A., Buntinx, W. H. E. *et al.* (2002). *Mental Retardation: Definition, Classification, and Systems of Supports.* 10th edn. Washington, DC: American Association on Mental Retardation.

Lucyshyn, J. M., Olson, D. and Horner, R. H. (1995). Building an ecology of support: a case study of one young woman with severe problem behaviors living in the community. *Journal of the Association For Persons With Severe Handicaps*, **20**, 16–30.

Lucyshyn, J. M., Kayser, A. T., Irvin, L. K. and Blumberg, E. R. (2002). Functional assessment and positive behavior support at home with families: designing effective and contextually appropriate behavior support plans. In J. M. Lucyshyn, G. Dunlap and R. W. Albin, eds. *Families and Positive Behavior Support.* Baltimore: Brookes.

Luiselli, J. K. (1992). Protective equipment. In J. K. Luiselli, J. L. Matson and N. N. Singh, eds. *Self Injurious Behavior: Analysis, Assessment and Treatment.* New York: Springer Verlag.

Luiselli, J. K. (2006). *Antecedent Assessment and Intervention: Supporting Children and Adults with Developmental Disabilities in Community Settings.* Baltimore Brookes.

Luiselli, J. K. (2009). Physical restraint of people with intellectual disability: a review of implementation reduction and elimination procedures. *Journal of Applied Research in Intellectual Disabilities*, **22**, 126–134.

Lundahl, B., Risser, H. J. and Lovejoy, M. C. (2006). A meta-analysis of parent training: Moderators and follow-up effects. *Clinical Psychology Review*, **26**, 86–104.

Lundstrom, M., Astrom, S. and Granheim, U. H. (2007). Caregivers' experiences of exposure to violence in services for people with learning disabilities. *Journal of Psychiatric and Mental Health Nursing*, **14**, 338–345.

Luthar, S., Sawyer, J. and Brown, P. (2006). Conceptual issues in studies of resilience. Past, present, and future research. *Annals of the New York Academy of Sciences*, **1094**, 105–115.

Luthar, S. S. (2003). *Resilience and Vulnerability: Adaptation in the Context of Childhood Adversities.* Cambridge: Cambridge University Press.

Luthar, S. S. (2006). Resilience in development: a synthesis of research across five decades. In D. Cicchetti and D. J. Cohen, eds. *Developmental Psychopathology, Vol 3: Risk, Disorder, and Adaptation.* Hoboken, NJ: John Wiley & Sons.

Luthar, S. S. and Brown, P. J. (2007). Maximizing resilience through diverse levels of inquiry: prevailing paradigms, possibilities, and priorities for the future. *Development and Psychopathology*, **19**, 931–955.

Luthar, S. S., Cicchetti, D. and Becker, B. (2000). The construct of resilience: a critical evaluation and guidelines for future work. *Child Development*, **71**, 543–562.

Lynch, J. W., Kaplan, G. A. and Shema, S. J. (1997). Cumulative impact of sustained economic hardship on physical, cognitive, psychological, and social functioning. *The New England Journal of Medicine*, **337**, 1889–1895.

Mace, F. C. (1994). Basic research needed for stimulating the development of behavioral technologies. *Journal of the Experimental Analysis of Behavior*, **61**, 529–550.

Mace, F. C. and Knight, D. (1986). Functional analysis and treatment of severe pica. *Journal of Applied Behavior Analysis*, **19**, 411–416.

Mace, F. C. and Belfiore, P. (1990). Behavioral momentum in the treatment of escape-motivated stereotypy. *Journal of Applied Behavior Analysis*, **23**, 507–514.

Mace, F. C. and Lalli, J. S. (1991). Linking descriptive and experimental analyses in the treatment of bizarre speech. *Journal of Applied Behavior Analysis*, **24**, 553–562.

Mace, F. C. and Roberts, M. L. (1993). Factors affecting selection of behavioral interventions. In J. Reichle and D. P. Wacker, eds. *Communicative Alternatives to Challenging Behavior*. Baltimore: Brookes.

Mace, F. C., Hock, M. L., Lalli, J. S. *et al.* (1988). Behavioral momentum in the treatment of noncompliance. *Journal of Applied Behavior Analysis*, **21**, 123–141.

Mace, F. C., Yankanich, M. A. and West, B. (1989). Toward a methodology of experimental analysis and treatment of aberrant classroom behaviors. *Special Services in the School*, **4**, 71–88.

Mace, F. C., Lalli, J. S. and Lalli, E. P. (1991). Functional analysis and treatment of aberrant behavior. *Research in Developmental Disabilities*, **12**, 155–180.

Machalicek, W., O'Reilly, M. F., Beretvas, N., Sigafoos, J. and Lancioni, G. E. (2008). A review of interventions to reduce challenging behavior in school settings for students with autism spectrum disorders. *Research in Autistic Spectrum Disorders*, **2**, 395–416.

MacLean, W. E., Stone, W. L. and Brown, W. H. (1994). Developmental psychopathology of destructive behavior. In T. Thompson and D. B. Gray, eds. *Destructive Behavior in Developmental Disabilities: Diagnosis and Treatment*. Thousand Oaks: Sage.

Maiano, C., Ninot, G. and Errais, B. (2001). Effects of alternate sport competition in perceived competence for adolescent males with mild to moderate mental retardation. *International Journal of Rehabilitation Research*, **24**, 51–58.

Mansell, J. (1995). Staffing and staff performance in services for people with severe or profound learning disability and seriously challenging behaviour. *Journal of Intellectual Disability Research*, **39**, 3–14.

Mansell, J., McGill, P. and Emerson, E. (2001). Development and evaluation of innovative residential services for people with severe intellectual disability and serious challenging behaviour. In L. M. Glidden, ed. *International Review of Research in Mental Retardation*. New York: Academic Press.

Marmot, M. and Wilkinson, R. G. (2006). *Social Determinants of Health*. Oxford: Oxford University Press.

Marquis, J. G., Horner, R. H., Carr, E. G. *et al.* (2000). A meta-analysis of positive behaviour support. In R. Gersten, E. P. Schiller and S. Vaughn, eds. *Contemporary Special Education Research*. New York: Lawrence Erlbaum Associates.

Martens, B. K., DiGennaro, F. D., Reed, D. D., Szczech, F. M. and Rosenthal, B. D. (2008). Contingency space analysis: An alternative method for identifying contingent relations from observational data. *Journal of Applied Behavior Analysis*, **41**, 69–81.

Martorell, A., Gutierrez-Recacha, P., Pereda, A. and Ayuso-Mateos, J. L. (2008). Identification of personal factors that determine work outcome for adults with intellectual disability. *Journal of Intellectual Disability Research*, **52**, 1091–1101.

Mason, T. (1996). Seclusion and learning disabilities: Research and deduction. *British Journal of Developmental Disabilities*, **17**, 149–159.

Masters, K. J. (2008). Modernizing seclusion and restraint. In M. Nunno, D. Day and L. Bullard, eds. *Examining the Safety of High-risk Interventions for Children and Young People*. New York: Child Welfare League of America.

Matson, J. L. and Minshawi, N. F. (2007). Functional assessment of challenging behavoir: toward a strategy for applied settings. *Research in Developmental Disabilities*, **2007**, 353–361.

Matson, J. L. and Nebel-Schwalm, M. (2007). Assessing challenging behaviors in children with autism spectrum disorders: a review. *Research in Developmental Disabilities*, **28**, 567–579.

Matson, J. L. and Neal, D. (2009). Psychotropic medication use for challenging behaviors in persons with intellectual disabilities: an overview. *Research in Developmental Disabilities*, **30**, 572–586.

Matson, J. L., Bamburg, J. W., Cherry, K. E. and Paclawskyj, T. R. (1999). A validity study on the Questions About Behavioral Function (QABF) scale: predicting treatment success for self-injury, aggression and stereotypies. *Research in Developmental Disabilities*, **20**, 163–176.

Matson, J. L., Fodstad, J. C., Neal, D., Dempsey, T. and Rivet, T. T. (2010). Risk factors for tardive dyskinesia in adults with intellectual disability, comorbid pathology, and long-term psychtropic use. *Research in Developmental Disabilities*, **31**, 108–116.

Matthews, T., Weston, N., Baxter, H., Felce, D. and Kerr, M. (2008). A general practice-based prevalence study of epilepsy among adults with intellectual disabilities and of its association with psychiatric disorder, behaviour disturbance and carer stress. *Journal of Intellectual Disability Research*, **52**, 163–173.

Maughan, B., Rowe, R., Messer, J., Goodman, R. and Meltzer, H. (2004). Conduct disorder and oppositional defiant disorder in a national sample: developmental epidemiology. *Journal of Child Psychology and Psychiatry*, **45**, 609–621.

Maurice, P. and Trudel, G. (1982). Self injurious behavior: Prevalence and relationships to environmental events. In J. H. Hollis and C. E. Meyers, eds. *Life Threatening Behavior: Analysis and Intervention*. Washington, DC: American Association on Mental Deficiency.

McAfee, J. K. (1987). Classroom density and the aggressive behavior of handicapped children. *Education and Treatment of Children*, **10**, 134–145.

McAtee, M., Carr, E. G. and Schulte, C. (2004). A contextual assessment inventory for problem behavior: initial development. *Journal of Positive Behavior Interventions*, **6**, 148–165.

McComas, J., Moore, T., Dahl, N., Hartman, E., Hoch, J. and Symons, F. (2009). Calculating contingencies in natural environments: Issues in the application of sequential analysis. *Journal of Applied Behavior Analysis*, **42**, 413–423.

McConachie, H. and Diggle, T. (2007). Parent implemented early intervention for young children with autism spectrum disorder: a systematic review. *Journal of Evaluation in Clinical Practice*, **13**, 120–129.

McDonald, W. and Viehbeck, S. (2007). From evidence-based practice making to practice-based evidence making: creating communities of (research) and practice. *Health Promotion Practice*, **8**, 140–144.

McDonnell, A. (2009). The effectiveness of training in physical intervention. In D. Allen, ed. *Ethical Approaches to Physical Interventions. Volume 2.* Kidderminster: BILD Publications.

McDonnell, A. and Sturmey, P. (2000). The social validation of physical restraint procedures with people with developmental disabilities: a comparison of young people and professional groups. *Research in Developmental Disabilities*, **21**, 85–92.

McDonnell, A., Dearden, B. and Richens, A. (1991). Staff training in the management of violence and aggression. 1-Setting up a training system. *Mental Handicap* **19**, 73–76.

McDonnell, A., Sturmey, P. and Dearden, B. (1993). The acceptability of physical restraint procedures for people with a learning difficulty. *Behavioural and Cognitive Psychotherapy*, **21**, 255–264.

McDowell, J. J. (1982). The importance of Herrnstein's mathematical statement of the law of effect for behavior therapy. *American Psychologist*, **37**, 771–779.

McGill, P. (1999). Establishing operations: implications for the assessment, treatment, and prevention of problem behavior. *Journal of Applied Behavior Analysis*, **32**, 393–418.

McGill, P., Murphy, G. and Kelly-Pike, A. (2009). Frequency of use and characteristics of people with intellectual disabilities subject to physical interventions. *Journal of Applied Research in Intellectual Disabilities*, **22**, 152–158.

McIntyre, L. L. (2008a). Adapting Webster–Stratton's Incredible Years parent training programme for children with developmental delay: findings from a treatment group only study. *Journal of Intellectual Disability Research*, **52**, 1176–1192.

McIntyre, L. L. (2008b). Parent training for young children with developmental disabilities: randomized controlled trial. *American Journal of Mental Retardation*, **113**, 356–368.

McLean, G. and Grey, I. (2007). Modifying challenging behaviour and planning positive supports. In A. Carr, G. O'Reilly, P. N. Walsh and J. McEvoy, eds. *The Handbook of Intellectual Disability and Clinical Practice*. London: Routledge.

McLeod, J. D. and Shanahan, M. J. (1996). Trajectories of poverty and children's mental health. *Journal of Health and Social Behavior*, **37**, 207–220.

Mental Health Act Commission (2006). *In Place of Fear? Eleventh Biennial Report*. London: TSO.

Mental Health Foundation (1997). *Don't Forget Us: Children With Learning Disabilities and Severe Challenging Behaviour*. London: Mental Health Foundation.

Mercy, J. A. and Saul, J. (2009). Creating a healthier furtur through early interventions for children. *Journal of the American Medical Association*, **301**, 2262–2264.

Merrell, K. W. and Holland, M. L. (1997). Social emotional behavior of preschool-age children with and without developmental delays. *Research in Developmental Disabilities*, **18**, 393–405.

Meyer, L. H. and Janney, R. (1989). User friendly measures of meaningful outcomes: evaluating behavioral interventions. *Journal of the Association for Persons with Severe Handicaps*, **14**, 262–270.

Meyer, L. H. and Evans, I. M. (1993). Meaningful outcomes in behavioral intervention: evaluating positive approaches to the remediation of challenging behaviors. In J. Reichle and D. P. Wacker, eds. *Communicative Alternatives to Challenging Behavior*. Baltimore: Paul H Brookes.

Michael, J. (1982). Distinguishing between discriminative and motivational functions of stimuli. *Journal of the Experimental Analysis of Behavior*, **37**, 149–155.

Michael, J. (1993). Establishing operations. *The Behavior Analyst*, **16**, 191–206.

Michael, J. (2000). Implications and refinements of the establishing operation concept. *Journal of Applied Behavior Analysis*, **33**, 401–410.

Mihalopoulos, C., Sanders, M. R., Turner, K. M. T., Murphy-Brennan, M. and Carter, R. (2007). Does the triple-positive parenting program provide value for money? *Australian and New Zealand Journal of Psychiatry*, **41**, 239–246.

Miller, J. A., Hunt, D. P. and Georges, M. A. (2006). Reduction of physical restraints in residential treatment facilities. *Journal of Disability Policy Studies*, **16**, 202–208.

Miltenberger, R. G. (2006). Antecedent interventions for challenging behaviors maintained by escape from instructional activities. In J. K. Luiselli, ed. *Antecedent Assessment and Intervention*, Baltimore: Paul H Brookes.

Mohr, W. K., Petti, T. A. and Mohr, B. B. (2003). Adverse effects associated with physical restraint. *Canadian Journal of Psychiatry*, **48**, 330–337.

Monaghan, M. T. and Soni, S. (1992). Effects of significant life events on the behaviour of mentally handicapped people in the community. *British Journal of Mental Subnormality*, **38**, 114–121.

Morris, E. K. and Midgley, B. D. (1990). Some historical and conceptual foundations of ecobehavioral analysis. In S. R. Schroeder, ed. *Ecobehavioral Analysis and Developmental Disabilities*. New York: Springer–Verlag.

Moss, S., Emerson, E., Kiernan, C., Turner, S., Hatton, C. and Alborz, A. (2000). Psychiatric symptoms in adults with learning disability and challenging behaviour. *British Journal of Psychiatry*, **177**, 452–456.

Murphy, C. M., Boyle, C., Schendel, D., Decoufle, P. and Yeargin-Allsop, M. (1988). Epidemiology of mental retardation in children. *Mental Retardation and Developmental Disabilities Research Reviews*, **4**, 6–13.

Murphy, G., Eilsien, D. and Clare, I. (1996). Services for people with mild intellectual disabilities and challenging behaviour. *Journal of Applied Research in Intellectual Disabilities*, **9**, 256–283.

Murphy, G., Kelly-Pike, A. and McGill, P. (2002). Assessing the impact of the BILD/NAS initiative. In D. Allen, ed. *Ethical Approaches to Physical Intervention. Responding to Challenging Behaviour in People with Intellectual Disabilities*. Kidderminster: BILD Publications.

Murphy, G. H., Oliver, C., Corbett, J. *et al*. (1993). Epidemiology of self injury, characteristics of people with severe self injury and initial treatment outcome. In C. Kiernan, ed. *Research to Practice? Implications of Research on the Challenging Behaviour of People with Learning Disabilities*. Kidderminster: BILD.

Murphy, G. H., Hall, S., Oliver, C. and Kissi-Debra, R. (1999a). Identification of early self-injurious behaviour in young children with intellectual disability. *Journal of Intellectual Disability Research*, **43**, 149–163.

Murphy, G. H., O'Callaghan, A. C. and Clare, I. C. H. (2007). The impact of alleged abuse on behaviour in adults with severe intellectual disabilities. *Journal of Intellectual Disability Research*, **51**, 741–749.

Murphy, K. C., Jones, L. A. and Owen, M. J. (1999b). High rates of schizophrenia in adults with velo-cardio-facial syndrome. *Archives of General Psychiatry*, **56**, 940–945.

Nagin, D. and Tremblay, R. E. (1999). Trajectories of boys' physical aggression, opposition, and hyperactivity on the path to physically violent and non violent juvenile delinquency. *Child Development*, **70**, 1181–1196.

National Institute for Clinical Excellence (2005). *Violence. The Short-term Management of Disturbed/Violent Behaviour in In-patient Psychiatric Settings and Emergency Departments*. London: Royal College of Nursing.

National Taskforce on Violence Against Social Care Staff (2000). *Violence against Social Care Staff. Qualitative Research*. London: Research Perspectives.

Netto, G., Bhopal, R., Lederle, N., Khatoon, J. and Jackson, A. (2010). How can health promotion interventions be adapted for minority ethnic communities? Five principles for guiding the development of behavioural interventions. *Health Promotion International*, **25**, 248–257.

Newton, J. T. and Sturmey, P. (1991). The Motivation Assessment Scale: inter rater reliability and internal consistency in a British sample. *Journal of Mental Deficiency Research*, **35**, 472–474.

Ninot, G., Bilard, J. and Delignières, D. (2005). Effects of integrated or segregated sport participation on the physical self for adolescents with intellectual disabilities. *Journal of Intellectual Disability Research*, **49**, 682–689.

Noone, S. P. and Hastings, R. P. (in press). Building psychological resilience in support staff caring for people with intellectual disabilities: pilot evaluation of an acceptance-based intervention. *Journal of Applied Research in Intellectual Disabilities*.

Northup, J., Wacker, D. P., Sasso, G. *et al.* (1991). A brief functional analysis of aggressive and alternative behavior in an out clinic setting. *Journal of Applied Behavior Analysis*, **24**, 509–522.

Nunno, M. A., Holden, M. J. and Tollar, A. (2006). Learning from tragedy: a survey of child and adolescent restraint fatalities. *Child Abuse and Neglect*, **30**, 1333–1342.

NYS Commission on Quality of Care for the Mentally Disabled (1994). *Voices from the front line. In Patients' Perspectives of Restraint and Seclusion Use*. New York: Commission on Quality of Care for the Mentally Disabled.

O'Neill, R. E., Horner, R. H., Albin, R. W., Storey, K. and Sprague, J. R. (1997). *Functional Analysis and Program Development For Problem behavior*. Pacific Grove: Brooks/Cole.

O'Reilly, M. F. (1995). Functional analysis and treatment of escape-maintained aggression correlated with sleep deprivation. *Journal of Applied Behavior Analysis*, **28**, 225–226.

O'Reilly, M. F. (1996). Assessment and treatment of episodic self-injury: a case study. *Research in Developmental Disabilities*, **17**, 349–361.

O'Reilly, M. F., Lancioni, G. E. and Emerson, E. (1999). A systematic analysis of the influence of prior social context on aggression and self-injury within analogue analysis assessments. *Behavior Modification*, **23**: 4, 578–596.

O'Reilly, M. F., Cannella, H., Sigafoos, J. and Lancioini, G. E. (2006). Communication and social skills interventions. In J. K. Luiselli, ed. *Antecedent Assessment and Intervention*. Baltimore: Paul H Brookes.

O'Reilly, M. F., Sigafoos, J., Lancioni, G. E. *et al.* (2007). Applied behaviour analysis. In A. Carr, G. O'Reilly, P. N. Walsh and J. McEvoy, eds. *The Handbook of Intellectual Disability and Clinical Psychology Practice*. London: Routledge.

Offord, D. R. and Bennett, K. J. (2002). Prevention. In M. Rutter and E. Taylor, eds. *Child and Adolescent Psychiatry*. Oxford: Blackwell.

Oliver, C. (1993). Self injurious behaviour: from response to strategy. In C. Kiernan, ed. *Research to Practice? Implication of Research on the Challenging Behaviour of People with Learning Disabilities*. Clevedon: British Institute of Learning Disabilities.

Oliver, C., Murphy, G. H. and Corbett, J. A. (1987). Self injurious behaviour in people with mental handicap: a total population survey. *Journal of Mental Deficiency Research*, **31**, 147–162.

Oliver, C., Hall, S. and Murphy, G. (2005). The early development of self-injurious behaviour: evaluating the role of social reinforcement. *Journal of Intellectual Disability Research*, **49**, 591–599.

Owen, D. M., Hastings, R. P., Noone, S. J., Chinn, J., Harman, K. and Roberts, J. (2004). Life events as correlates of problem behavior and mental health in a residential population of adults with developmental disabilities. *Research in Developmental Disabilities*, **25**, 309–320.

Parish, S. L., Rose, R. A., Andrews, M. E., Grinstein-Weiss, M. and Richman, E. L. (2008). Material hardship in US families raising children with disabilities. *Exceptional Children*, **75**, 71–92.

Parkes, B. A. and Carson, R. (2008). Sudden death during restraint: do some positions affect lung function? *Medicine, Science and Law*, **48**, 137–141.

Parrish, J. M., Cataldo, M. F., Kolko, D. J., Neef, N. A. and Egel, A. L. (1986). Experimental analysis of response covariation among compliant and inappropriate behaviors. *Journal of Applied Behavior Analysis*, **19**, 241–254.

Parrish, J. M. and Roberts, M. L. (1993). Interventions based on covariation of desired and inappropriate behavior. In J. Reichle and D. P. Wacker, eds. *Communicative Alternatives to Challenging Behavior*. Baltimore: Paul H. Brookes.

Patel, V., Araya, R., Chatterjee, S. *et al.* (2007a). Treatment and prevention of mental disorders in low-income and middle-income countries. *Lancet*, **370**, 991–1005.

Patel, V., Flisher, A. J., Hetrick, S. and McGorry, P. (2007b). Mental health of young people: a global public-health challenge. *Lancet*, **369**, 1302–1313.

Paterson, B., Leadbetter, D., Miller, G. and Crichton, J. (2008). Adopting a public health model to reduce violence and restraints in children's residential facilities. In M. Nunno, D. Day and L. Bullard, eds. *Examining the Safety of High-risk Interventions for Children and Young People*. New York: Child Welfare League of America.

Paterson, B. A., Bradley, P., Stark, C., Saddler, D., Leadbetter, D. and Allen, D. (2003). Deaths associated with restraint use in health and social care in the UK. The results of a preliminary survey. *Journal of Psychiatric and Mental Health Nursing*, **10**, 3–15.

Patterson, G. R. and Reid, J. B. (1984). Social interactional processes within the family: the study of the moment-by-moment family transactions in which human social development is embedded. *Journal of Applied Developmental Psychology*, **5**, 237–262.

Peck, S. M., Wacker, D. P., Berg, W. K. *et al.* (1996). Choice-making treatment of young children's severe behavior problems. *Journal of Applied Behavior Analysis*, **29**, 263–290.

Peine, H. A., Darvish, R., Adams, K., Blalelock, H., Jenson, W. and Osborne, J. G. (1995). Medical problems, maladaptive behaviors and the developmentally disabled. *Behavioral Interventions*, **10**, 149–160.

Pence, S. T., Roscoe, E. M., Bourret, J. C. and Ahearn, W. H. (2009). Relative contributions of three descriptive methods: Implications for behavioral assessment. *Journal of Applied Behavior Analysis*, **42**, 425–446.

Perry, D., Shervington, T., Mungur, N., Marston, G., Martin, D. and Brown, G. (2007). Why are people with intellectual disability moved "out-of-area"? *Journal of Policy and Practice in Intellectual Disabilities*, **4**, 203–209.

Petitclerc, A. and Tremblay, R. E. (2009). Childhood disruptive behaviour disorders: review of their origin, development and prevention. *The Canadian Journal of Psychiatry*, **54**, 222–231.

Petterson, S. M. and Albers, A. B. (2004). Effects of poverty and maternal depression on early child development. *Child Development*, **72**, 1794–1813.

Piazza, C. C., Hagopian, L. P., Hughes, C. R. and Fisher, W. W. (1998). Using chronotherapy to treat severe sleep problems: a case study. *American Journal of Mental Retardation*, **102**, 358–366.

Plant, K. M. and Sanders, M. R. (2007). Reducing problem behavior during care-giving in families of preschool-aged children with developmental disabilities. *Research in Developmental Disabilities*, **28**, 362–385.

Plomin, R., Price, T. S., Eley, T. C., Dale, P. S. and Stevenson, J. (2002). Associations between behaviour problems and verbal and nonverbal cognitive abilities and disabilities in early childhood. *Journal of Child Psychology and Psychiatry*, **43**, 619–633.

Podboy, J. W. and Mallery, W. A. (1977). Caffeine reduction and behavior change in the severely retarded. *Mental Retardation*, **15**, 40.

Pretscher, E. S., Rey, C. and Bailey, J. S. (2009). A review of empirical support for differential reinforcement of alternative behavior. *Research in Developmental Disabilities*, **30**, 409–425.

Prinz, R. J., Sanders, M. R., Shapiro, C. J., Whitaker, D. J. and Lutzker, J. R. (2009). Population-based prevention of child maltreatment. *Prevention Science*, **10**, 1–12.

Qureshi, H. (1990). Parents caring for young adults with mental handicap and behaviour problems. Manchester: Hester Adrian Research Centre, University of Manchester.

Qureshi, H. (1994). The size of the problem. In E. Emerson, P. McGill and J. Mansell, eds. *Severe Learning Disabilities and Challenging Behaviours: Designing High Quality Services*. London: Chapman & Hall.

Qureshi, H. and Alborz, A. (1992). The epidemiology of challenging behaviour. *Mental Handicap Research*, **5**, 130–145.

Ramey, C. T. and Ramey, S. L. (1998). Early intervention and early experience. *American Psychologist*, **53**, 109–120.

Rangecroft, M. E., Tyrer, S. P. and Berney, T. P. (1997). The use of seclusion and emergency medication in a hospital for people for people with learning disability. *British Journal of Psychiatry*, **170**, 273–277.

Rast, J., Johnston, J. M., Drum, C. and Conrin, J. (1981). The relation of food quantity to rumination behavior. *Journal of Applied Behavior Analysis*, **14**, 121–130.

Rast, J., Johnston, J. M. and Drum, C. (1984). A parametric analysis of the relationship between food quantity and rumination. *Journal of the Experimental Analysis of Behavior*, **41**, 125–134.

Reid, A. H. and Ballinger, B. R. (1995). Behaviour symptoms among severely and profoundly mentally retarded patients. *British Journal of Psychiatry*, **167**, 452–455.

Reid, D. H., Iverson, J. M. and Green, C. W. (1999). A systematic evaluation of preferences identified through person-centred planning for people with profound multiple disabilities. *Journal of Applied Behavior Analysis*, **32**, 467–478.

Reiss, S. and Aman, M. (1998). *Psychotropic Medication and Developmental Disabilities: The International Consensus Handbook*. Ohio State University Nisonger Center.

Remington, B., Hastings, R. P., Kovshoff, H., Espinosa, F., Jahr, E. and Brown, T. (2007). Early intensive behavioral intervention: outcomes for children with autism and their parents after two years. *American Journal on Mental Retardation*, **112**, 418–438.

Repp, A. C. and Singh, N. N. (1990). *Perspectives on the Use of Nonaversive and Aversive Interventions for Persons with Developmental Disabilities*. Sycamore, Il: Sycamore Publishing Company.

Reynolds, A., Temple, J., Ou, S.-R. *et al.* (2007). Effects of a school-based, early childhood intervention on adult health and well-being: a 19-year follow up of low-income families. *Archives of Pediatric and Adolescent Medicine*, **161**, 730–733.

Ricciardi, J. N. (2006). Combining antecedent and consequence procedures in multi-component behavior support plans: a guide to writing plans with functional efficacy. In J. K. Luiselli, ed. *Antecedent Assessment and Intervention*. Baltimore: Paul H Brookes.

Richman, D. M. (2008). Early intervention and prevention of self-injurious behaviour exhibited by young children with developmental disabilities. *Journal of Intellectual Disability Research*, **52**: 1, 3–17.

Richman, D. M. and Lindauer, S. E. (2005). Longitudinal assessment of stereotypic, proto-injurious and self-injurious behavior exhibited by young children with developmental delays. *American Journal on Mental Retardation*, **110**, 439–450.

Richman, D. M., Wacker, D. P., Asmus, J. M. and Casey, S. D. (1998). Functional analysis and extinction of different behavior problems exhibited by the same individual. *Journal of Applied Behavior Analysis*, **31**, 475–478.

Richman, D. M., Wacker, D. P., Asmus, J. M., Casey, S. D. and Andelman, M. (1999). Further analysis of problem behavior in response class hierarchies. *Journal of Applied Behavior Analysis*, **32**, 269–283.

Richter, D., Needham, I. and Kunz, S. (2006). The effects of aggression management training for mental health care and disability staff: a systematic review. In D. Richter and R. Whittington, eds. *Violence in Health Settings. Causes, Consequences, Management*. New York: Springer.

Rinck, C. (1998). Epidemiology and psychoactive medication. In S. Reiss and M. G. Aman, eds. *Psychotropic Medication and Developmental Disabilities: The International Consensus Handbook*. Ohio: Nisonger Center, Ohio State University.

Rincover, A. and Devany, J. (1982). The application of sensory extinction procedures to self injury. *Analysis and Intervention in Developmental Disabilities*, **2**, 67–81.

Ringdahl, J. E., Vollmer, T. R., Marcus, B. A. and Roane, H. S. (1997). An analogue evaluation of environmental enrichment: the role of stimulus preference. *Journal of Applied Behavior Analysis*, **30**, 203–216.

Risley, T. (1996). Get a life! Positive behavioral intervention for challenging behavior through life arrangement and life coaching. In L. K. Koegel, R. L. Koegel and G. Dunlap, eds. *Positive Behavioral Support: Including People With Difficult Behavior in the Community*. Baltimore: Paul H Brookes.

Roberts, C., Mazzucchelli, T., Studman, L. and Sanders, M. R. (2006). Behavioural family intervention for children with developmental disabilities and behavioural problems. *Journal of Clinical Child and Adolescent Psychology*, **35**, 180–193.

Robertson, J., Emerson, E., Gregory, N., Hatton, C., Kessissoglou, S. and Hallam, A. (2000). Receipt of psychotropic medication by people with intellectual disability in residential settings. *Journal of Intellectual Disability Research*, **44**, 666–676.

Robertson, J., Emerson, E., Gregory, N. *et al.* (2001a). Social networks of people with mental retardation in residential settings. *Mental Retardation*, **39**, 201–214.

Robertson, J., Emerson, E., Hatton, C. *et al.* (2001b). Environmental opportunities and supports for exercising self-determination in community-based residential settings. *Research in Developmental Disabilities*, **22**: 6, 487–502.

Robertson, J., Emerson, E., Pinkney, L. *et al.* (2005). Treatment and management of challenging behaviour in congregate and noncongregate community-based supported accommodation. *Journal of Intellectual Disability Research*, **49**, 63–72.

Robertson, J., Emerson, E., Hatton, C. and Yasamy, M. T. (2009a). The efficacy of community-based rehabilitation for children with or at significant risk of intellectual disabilities in low and middle income countries : a review. Lancaster: Centre for Disability Research, Lancaster University.

Robertson, J., Hatton, C., Emerson, E. and Yasamy, M. T. (2009b). The identification of children with or at significant risk of intellectual disabilities in low and middle income countries: a review. Lancaster: Centre for Disability Research, Lancaster University.

Roeleveld, N., Zielhuis, G. A. and Gabreels, F. (1997). The prevalence of mental retardation: a critical review of recent literature. *Developmental Medicine and Child Neurology*, **39**, 125–132.

Rogers, P., Ghroum, P., Benson, R., Forward, L. and Gournay, K. (2006). Is breakaway training effective? An audit of one secure unit. *Journal of Forensic Psychiatry and Psychology*, **17**, 593–602.

Rojahn, J. (1994). Epidemiology and topographic taxonomy of self injurious behavior. In T. Thompson and D. B. Gray (eds.), *Destructive Behavior in Developmental Disabilities: Diagnosis and Treatment*. Thousand Oaks: Sage.

Rojahn, J. and Marshburn, E. C. (1992). Facial screening and visual occlusion. In J. K. Luiselli, J. K. Matson and N. N. Singh, eds. *Self-Injurious Behavior: Analysis, Assessment and Treatment*. New York: Springer-Verlag.

Rojahn, J. and Esbensen, A. J. (2002). Epidemiology of self-injurious behavior in mental retardation: a review. In S. R. Schroeder, M. L. Oster-Granite and T. Thompson, eds. *Self-Injurious Behavior: Gene–Brain–Behavior Relationships*. Washington, DC: American Psychological Association.

Rolider, A. and Van Houten, R. (1990). The role of reinforcement in reducing inappropriate behavior: some myths and misconceptions. In A. C. Repp and N. N. Singh, eds.

Perspectives on the Use of Nonaversive and Aversive Interventions for Persons with Developmental Disabilities. Sycamore, IL: Sycamore.

Romanczyk, R. G. and Matthews, A. J. (1998). Physiological state as antecedent: utilization in functional analysis. In J. Luiselli and M. J. Cameron, eds. *Antecedent Control: Innovative Approaches to Behavioral Support.* Baltimore: Brookes.

Romanczyk, R. G., Lockshin, S. and O'Connor, J. (1992). Psychophysiology and issues of anxiety and arousal. In J. Luiselli, J. L. Matson and N. N. Singh, eds. *Self Injurious Behavior: Analysis, Assessment and Treatment.* New York: Springer-Verlag.

Romeo, R., Knapp, M., Tyrer, P., Crawford, M. and Oliver-Africano, P. (2009). The treatment of challenging behaviour in intellectual disabilities: cost-effectiveness analysis. *Journal of Intellectual Disability Research*, **53**, 633–643.

Rosales-Ruiz, J. and Baer, D. M. (1997). Behavioral cusps: a developmental and pragmatic concept for behavior analysis. *Journal of Applied Behavior Analysis*, **30**, 533–544.

Roscoe, E. M., Iwata, B. A. and Goh, H.-L. (1998). A comparison of noncontingent reinforcement and sensory extinction as treatments for self-injurious behavior. *Journal of Applied Behavior Analysis*, **31**, 635–646.

Rose, S. and Massey, P. (1993). Adventurous outdoor activities: an investigation into the benefits of adventure for seven people with severe learning difficulties. *Mental Handicap Research*, **6**, 287–302.

Rowett, C. and Breakwell, G. (1992). *Managing Violence at Work. A Course Leader's Guide.* Windsor: NFER Nelson.

Royal College of Psychiatrists (1995). Strategies for the management of disturbed and violent patients in psychiatric units: council report CR41, London: Royal College of Psychiatrists.

Royal College of Psychiatrists, British Psychological Society and Royal College of Speech and Language Therapists (2007). Clinical and service guidelines for supporting people with learning disabilities who are at risk of receiving abusive or restrictive practices. London: Royal College of Psychiatrists.

Rusch, R., Hall, J. C. and Griffin, H. (1986). Abuse provoking characteristics of institutionalized mentally retarded individuals. *American Journal of Mental Deficiency*, **90**, 618–624.

Rutter, M. (1979). Protective factors in children's responses to stress and disadvantage. In M. W. Kent and J. E. Rolf, eds. *Primary Prevention of Psychopathology. III. Social Competence in Children.* Hanover, NH: University Press of New England.

Rutter, M. (1985). Resilience in the face of adversity: protective factors and resistence to psychiatric disorders. *British Journal of Psychiatry*, **147**, 589–611.

Rutter, M. (1987). Psychosocial resilience and protective mechanisms. *American Journal of Orthopsychiatry*, **57**, 316–331.

Rutter, M. (1999). Resilience concepts and findings: implications for family therapy. *Journal of Family Therapy*, **21**, 119–44.

Rutter, M. (2000). Psychosocial influences: critiques, findings, and research needs. *Developmental Psychopathology*, **12**, 119–144.

Rutter, M., Bishop, D., Pine, D. *et al.* (2008). *Rutter's Child and Adolescent Psychiatry.* Oxford: Blackwell.

Sailas, E. and Fenton, M. (1999). Seclusion and restraint for serious mental illness. *Cochrane Database of Systematic Reviews*, **4**.

Samaha, A. L., Vollmer, T. R., Borrero, C., Sloman, K., Pipkin, C. and Bourret, J. (2009). Analyses of response-stimulus sequences in descriptive observations. *Journal of Applied Behavior Analysis*, 42, 447–468.

Sandberg, S. and Rutter, M. (2008). Acute life stresses. In M. Rutter, D. Bishop, D. Pine *et al.* eds. *Rutter's Child and Adolescent Psychiatry*. Oxford: Blackwell.

Sanders, K. (2009). The effects of an action plan, staff training, management support and monitoring on restraint use and costs of work related injuries. *Journal of Applied Research in Intellectual Disabilities*, 22, 216–222.

Sanders, M. R. (2008). Triple P-positive parenting program as a public health approach to strengthening parenting. *Journal of Family Psychology*, 22, 506–517.

Sanders, M. R. and Turner, K. M. T. (2002). The role of the media and primary care in the dissemination of evidence-based parenting and family support interventions. *Behavior Therapist*, 25, 156–166.

Sanders, M. R., Mazzucchelli, T. G. and Studman, L. J. (2004). Stepping stones triple P, *JIDD*, 29, 265–283.

Sandman, C. A., Touchette, P. E., Marion, S. D. and Chicz-DeMet, A. (2008). The role of proopiomelanocortin (POMC) in sequentially dependent self-injurious behavior. *Developmental Psychobiology*, 50, 680–689.

Saraceno, B., van Ommeren, M., Batniji, R. *et al.* (2007). Barriers to improvement of mental health services in low-income and middle-income countries. *Lancet*, 370, 1164–1174.

Saunders, R. R. and Saunders, M. D. (1998). Supported routines. In J. K. Luiselli and M. J. Cameron, eds. *Antecedent Control: Innovative Approaches to Behavioral Support*. Baltimore: Paul H Brookes.

Schalock, R. L. (1999). *Adaptive Behavior and Its Measurement*. Washington, DC: American Association on Mental Retardation.

Schalock, R. L. (2004). Adaptive behaviour: Its conceptualisation and measurement. In E. Emerson, C. Hatton, T. Thompson and T. Parmenter, eds. *International Handbook of Applied Research in Intellectual Disabilities*. Chichester: Wiley.

Schalock, R. L., Luckasson, R. A., Shogren, K. A. *et al.* (2007), The renaming of mental retardation: Understanding the change to the term intellectual disability. *Intellectual and Developmental Disabilities*, 45, 116–124.

Schoon, I. (2006). *Risk and Resilience: Adaptations in Changing Times*. Cambridge: Cambridge University Press.

Schreibman, L., Stahmer, A. C. and Pierce, K. L. (1996). Alternative applications of pivotal response training. In L. K. Koegel, R. L. Koegel and G. Dunlap, eds. *Positive Behavioral Support: Including People With Difficult Behavior in the Community*. Baltimore: Paul H Brookes.

Schroeder, S. R. and MacLean, W. (1987). If it isn't one thing it's another: experimental analysis of covariation in behavior management data of severe behavior disturbances. In S. Landesman and P. Vietze, eds. *Living Environments and Mental Retardation*. Washington, DC: American Association on Mental Retardation.

Schroeder, S. R. and Tessel, R. (1994). Dopaminergic and serotonergic mechanisms in self-injury and aggression. In T. Thompson and D. B. Gray, eds. *Destructive Behavior in Developmental Disabilities: Diagnosis and Treatment*. Thousand Oaks: Sage.

Schupf, N., Pang, D., Patel, B. N. *et al.* (2003). Onset of dementia is associated with age at menopause in women with Down's syndrome. *Annals of Neurology*, **54**: 4, 433–438.

Scotti, J. R. and Meyer, L. H. (1999). *Behavioral Intervention*. Baltimore: Brookes.

Scotti, J. R., Evans, I. M., Meyer, L. H. and DiBenedetto, A. (1991a). Individual repertoires as behavioural systems: Implications for program design and evaluation. In B. Remington, ed. *The Challenge of Severe Mental Handicap: A Behaviour Analytic Approach*. Chichester: Wiley.

Scotti, J. R., Evans, I. M. and Meyer, L. M. (1991b). A meta-analysis of intervention research with problem behaviour: treatment validity and standards of practice. *Journal of Intellectual Disability Research*, **96**, 233–256.

Scotti, J. R., Kimberley, J., Ujcich, K. L., Weigle, C. M., Holland, C. M. and Kirk, K. S. (1996). Interventions with challenging behavior of persons with developmental disabilities: a review of current research practices. *Journal of the Association for Persons with Severe Handicaps*, **21**, 123–134.

Seccombe, K. (2002). "Beating the Odds" versus "Changing the Odds": poverty, resilience, and family policy. *Journal of Marriage and the Family*, **64**, 384–394.

Seccombe, K. (2007). *Families in Poverty*. New York: Pearson Education.

Sequeira, H. and Halsted, S. (2001). "Is it meant to hurt, is it?" Management of violence in women with developmental disabilities. *Violence Against Women*, **7**, 462–476.

Sequeira, H. and Halstead, S. (2002). Control and restraint in the UK: service user perspectives. *British Journal of Forensic Practice*, **4**, 9–18.

Sequeira, H., Howlin, P. and Hollins, S. (2003). Psychological disturbance associated with sexual abuse in people with learning disabilities: case-control study. *British Journal of Psychiatry*, **183**, 451–456.

Severence, L. J. and Gastrom, L. L. (1977). Effects of the label 'mentally retarded' on causal explanations for success and failure outcomes. *American Journal on Mental Deficiency*, **81**, 547–555.

Shapira, N. A., Lessig, M. C., He, A. G., James, G. A., Driscoll, D. J. and Liu, Y. (2005). Satiety dysfunction in Prader–Willi syndrome demonstrated by fMRI. *Journal of Neurology, Neurosurgery and Psychiatry*, **76**: 2, 260–262.

Sigafoos, J. (1998). Choice making and personal selection strategies. In J. K. Luiselli and M. J. Cameron (eds.), *Antecedent Control: Innovative Approaches to Behavioral Support*. Baltimore: Paul H Brookes.

Sigafoos, J. (2000). Communication development and aberrant behavior in children with developmental disabilities. *Education and Training in Mental Retardation and Developmental Disabilities*, **35**, 168–176.

Sigafoos, J. and Kerr, M. (1994). Provision of leisure activities for the reduction of challenging behavior. *Behavioral Interventions*, **9**, 43–53.

Sigafoos, J. and Tucker, M. (2000). Brief assessment and treatment of multiple challenging behaviors. *Behavioral Interventions*, **15**, 53–70.

Sigafoos, J., Kerr, M. and Roberts, D. (1994). Interrater reliability of the Motivation Assessment Scale: failure to replicate with aggressive behavior. *Research in Developmental Disabilities*, **15**, 333–342.

Sigafoos, J., Arthur, M. and O'Reilly, M. (2003). *Challenging Behavior and Developmental Disability*. Baltimore: Brookes.

Sigafoos, J., O'Reilly, M. and Green, V. (2007). Communication difficulties and the promotion of communication skills. In A. Carr, G. O'Reilly, P. N. Walsh and J. McEvoy, eds. *The Handbook of Intellectual Disability and Clinical Psychology Practice*. New York: Routledge/Taylor & Francis.

Simmons, R. and Shiffman, J. (2007). Scaling up health service innovations: a framework for action. In R. Simmons, P. Fajans and L. Ghiron, eds. *Scaling up Health Service Delivery: From Pilot Innovations to Policies and Programmes*. Geneva: World Health Organization.

Singer, G. H., Goldberg-Hamblin, S. E., Peckham-Hardin, K. D., Barry, L. and Santarelli, G. E. (2002). Toward a synthesis of family support practices and positive behavior support. In J. M. Lucyshyn, G. Dunlap and R. W. Albin, eds. *Families and Positive Behavior Support*. Baltimore: Brookes.

Singh, A. N., Matson, J. L., Mouttapa, M., Pella, R. D., Hill, B. D. and Thorson, R. (2009a). A critical item analysis of the QABF: Development of a short form assessment instrument. *Research in Developmental Disabilities*, 30, 782–792.

Singh, N. N. and Repp, A. C. (1989). The behavioural and pharmacological management of problem behaviours in people with mental retardation. *Irish Journal of Psychology*, 9, 264–285.

Singh, N. N., Donatelli, L. S., Best, A. *et al.* (1993). Factor structure of the Motivation Assessment Schedule. *Journal of Intellectual Disability Research*, 37, 65–74.

Singh, N. N., Lancioini, G. E., Winton, A. S. W. *et al.* (2006a). Mindful staff increase learning and reduce aggression in adults with developmental disabilities. *Research in Developmental Disabilities*, 27, 345–358.

Singh, N. N., Winton, A. S. W., Singh, J., McAleavey, K., Wahler, R. G. and Sabaawi, M. (2006b). Mindfulness-based caregiving and support. In J. Luiselli, ed. *Antecedent Assessment and Intervention*, Baltimore: Paul H Brookes.

Singh, N. N., Lancioini, G. E., Winton, A. S. W., Singh, A. S., Askins, A. D. and Singh, J. (2009b). Mindful staff can reduce the use of physical restraints when providing care to individuals with intellectual disabilities. *Journal of Applied Research in Intellectual Disabilities*, 22, 194–202.

Skinner, B. F. (1966). An operant analysis of problem solving. In B. Klienmuntz, ed. *Problem Solving: Research, Methods and Theory*. New York: Wiley.

Smith, R. G. and Iwata, B. A. (1997). Antecedent influences on behavior disorders. *Journal of Applied Behavior Analysis*, 30, 343–375.

Snyder, R., Turgay, A., Aman, M. *et al.* (2002). Effects of risperidone on conduct and disruptive behavior disorders in children with subaverage IQs. *Journal of the American Academy of Child & Adolescent Psychiatry*, 41: 9, 1026–1036.

Society for Prevention Research (2004). *Standards of Evidence*. Falls Church: Society for Prevention Research.

Sohanpal, S. K., Deb, S., Thomas, C., Soni, R., Lenôtre, L. and Unwin, G. (2007). The effectiveness of antidepressant medication in the management of behaviour problems in adults with intellectual disabilities: a systematic review. *Journal of Intellectual Disability Research*, 51.

Solnick, J. V., Rincover, A. and Peterson, C. R. (1977). Some determinants of the reinforcing and punishing effects of timeout. *Journal of Applied Behavior Analysis*, 10, 415–424.

Spinelli, M., Rocha, A. C., Giacheti, C. M. and Richieri-Costa, A. (1995). Word-finding difficulties, verbal paraphasias, and verbal dyspraxia in ten individuals with fragile X syndrome. *American Journal of Medical Genetics*, **27**, 39–43.

Sprague, J. R. and Horner, R. H. (1992). Covariation within functional response classes: Implications for treatment of severe problem behavior. *Journal of Applied Behavior Analysis*, **25**, 735–745.

Spreat, S. and Connelly, L. (1996). Reliability analysis of the Motivation Assessment Scale. *American Journal on Mental Retardation*, **100**, 528–532.

Spreat, S., Conroy, J. W. and Fullerton, A. (2004). Statewide longitudinal survey of psychotropic medication use for persons with mental retardation: 1994 to 2000. *American Journal of Mental Retardation*, **109**, 322–331.

Staddon, J. E. R. (1977). Schedule induced behavior. In W. K. Honig and J. E. R. Staddon, eds. *Handbook of Operant Behavior*. Englewood Cliffs, NJ: Prentice Hall.

Stancliffe, R., Hayden, M. F. and Lakin, K. C. (1999). Effectiveness and quality of individual planning in residential settings: an analysis of outcomes. *Mental Retardation*, **37**, 104–116.

Steege, M. W., Wacker, D. P., Cigrand, K. C. *et al.* (1990). Use of negative reinforcement in the treatment of self-injurious behavior. *Journal of Applied Behavior Analysis*, **23**, 459–467.

Steen, P. L. and Zuriff, G. E. (1977). The use of relaxation in the treatment of self-injurious behavior. *Journal of Behavior Therapy and Experimental Psychiatry*, **8**, 447–448.

Steyaert, J., Legius, E., Borghgraef, M. and Fryns, J. (2003). A distinct neurocognitive phenotype in female fragile-X premutation carriers assessed with visual attention tasks. *American Journal of Medical Genetics Part A*, **116A 1**, 44–51.

Stuart, S. (2007). Communication disorders. In M. L. Batshaw, and N. J. Roizen, ed. *Children with Disabilities*, Baltimore: Brookes.

Stubbs, B., Leadbetter, D., Paterson, B., Yorston, G., Knight, C. and Davis, S. (2009) Physical interventions: a review of the literature on its use, staff and patient views, and the impact of training. *Journal of Psychiatric and Mental Health Nursing*, **16**, 99–105.

Sturmey, P. (1999). Correlates of restraint use in an institutional population. *Research in Developmental Disabilities*, **20**, 339–346.

Sturmey, P. (2009). Restraint, seclusion and PRN medication in English services for people with learning disabilities administered by the National Health Service: an analysis of the 2007 National Audit Survey. *Journal of Applied Research in Intellectual Disabilities*, **22**, 140–144.

Sturmey, P. and McGlyn, A. P. (2002). Restraint reduction. In D. Allen, ed. *Responding to Challenging Behaviour in Persons with Intellectual Disabilities: Ethical Approaches to Physical Intervention*. Kidderminster: British Institute of Learning Disabilities.

Sturmey, P., Lott, J. D., Laud, R. and Matson, J. L. (2005). Correlates of restraint use in an institutionalized population: a replication. *Journal of Intellectual Disability Research*, **49**, 501–506.

Symons, F. J., Clark, R. D., Hatton, D. D., Skinner, M. and Bailey Jr, D. B. (2003). Self-injurious behavior in young boys with fragile X syndrome. *American Journal of Medical Genetics Part A*, **118A: 2**, 115–121.

Symons, F. J., Thompson, T. and Rodriguez, M. C. (2004). Self-injurious behaviour and the efficacy of naltrexone treatment: a quantitative synthesis. *Mental Retardation and Developmental Disabilities Research Reviews*, **10**, 193–200.

Symons, F. J., Shinde, S. K. and Gilles, E. (2008). Perspectives on pain and intellectual disability. *Journal of Intellectual Disability Research*, **52**: Pt 4, 275–286.

Symons, F. J., Harper, V. N., McGrath, P. J., Breau, L. M. and Bodfish, J. W. (2009). Evidence of increased non-verbal signs of pain in adults with neurodevelopmental disorders and chronic self-injury. *Research in Developmental Disabilities*, **30**, 521–528.

Szymanski, L. and King, B. (1999). Summary of the practice parameters for the assessment and treatment of children, adolescents, and adults with mental retardation and comorbid mental disorders. *Journal of the American Academy of Child and Adolescent Psychiatry*, **38**, 1606–1610.

Talkington, L. and Riley, J. (1971). Reduction diets and aggression in institutionalized mentally retarded patients. *American Journal on Mental Deficiency*, **76**, 370–372.

Tate, B. G. and Baroff, G. S. (1966). Aversive control of self injurious behavior in a psychotic boy. *Behaviour Research and Therapy*, **4**, 281–287.

Tausig, M. (1985). Factors in family decision making about placement for developmentally disabled adults. *American Journal of Mental Deficiency*, **89**, 352–361.

Taylor, Oliver, C. and Murphy, G. (under review).

Taylor, D., Sandman, C. A., Touchette, P., Hetrick, W. P. and Barron, J. L. (1993a). Naltrexone improves learning and attention in self injurious individuals with developmental disabilities. *Journal of Developmental and Physical Disabilities*, **5**, 29–42.

Taylor, D. V., Rush, D., Hetrick, W. P. and Sandman, C. (1993b). Self injurious behavior within the menstrual cycle of women with mental retardation. *American Journal on Mental Retardation*, **97**, 659–664.

Taylor, J. C. and Carr, E. G. (1993). Reciprocal social influences in the analysis and intervention of severe challenging behavior. In J. Reichle and D. P. Wacker, eds. *Communicative Alternatives to Challenging Behavior*. Baltimore: Brookes.

Taylor, L. and Oliver, C. (2008). The behavioural phenotype of Smith–Magenis syndrome: evidence for a gene–environment interaction. *Journal of Intellectual Disability Research*, **52**, 830–841.

Thomas, R. and Zimmer-Gembeck, M. Z. (2007). Behavioral outcomes of parent–child interaction therapy and triple P-positive parenting program: a review and meta-analysis. *Journal of Abnormal Child Psychology*, **35**, 475–495.

Thompson, J. R., Bryant, B. R., Campbell, E. M. *et al.* (2004). *Supports Intensity Scale*. Washington, DC: American Association on Intellectual and Developmental Disabilities.

Thompson, R. W., Huefner, J. C., Vollmer, D. G., Davis, J. L. and Daly, D. L. (2008). A case study of organizational intervention to reduce physical interventions: creating effective, harm-free environments. In M. Nunno, D. Day and L. Bullard, eds. *Examining the Safety of High-risk Interventions for Children and Young People*. New York: Child Welfare League of America.

Thompson, S. and Emerson, E. (1995). Inter observer agreement on the Motivation Assessment Scale: another failure to replicate. *Mental Handicap Research*, **8**, 203–208.

Thompson, T. (2008). *Freedom from Meltdowns*. Baltimore: Brookes.

Thompson, T., Felce, D. and Symons, F. (2000). *Computer Assisted Behavioral Observation Methods for Developmental Disabilities*. Baltimore: Brookes.

Tilli, D. M. and Spreat, S. (2009) Restraint safety in a residential setting for persons with intellectual disabilities. *Behavioural Interventions*, 24, 127–136.

Tonge, B. J. and Einfeld, S. L. (2003). Psychopathology and intellectual disability. The Australian child to adult longitudinal study. *International Review of Research in Mental Retardation*, 26, 61–91.

Toogood, S. and Timlin, K. (1996). The functional assessment of challenging behaviour. *Journal of Applied Research in Intellectual Disabilities*, 9, 206–222.

Totsika, V. and Hastings, R. P. (2009). Persistent challenging behaviour in people with an intellectual disability. *Current Opinion in Psychiatry*, 22, 437–441.

Totsika, V., Toogood, A., Hastings, R. P. and Lewis, S. (2008). Persistence of challenging behaviours in adults with intellectual disability over a period of 11 years. *Journal of Intellectual Disability Research*, 52, 446–457.

Touchette, P. E., McDonald, R. F. and Langer, S. N. (1985). A scatter plot for identifying stimulus control of problem behavior. *Journal of Applied Behavior Analysis*, 18, 343–351.

Tremblay, R. E. (1999). When children's development fails. In D. P. Keating and C. Hertzman, eds. *Developmental Health and the Wealth of Nations: Social, Biological and Educational Dynamics*. New York: Guilford Press.

Tremblay, R. E. (2000). The development of aggressive behavior during childhood: What have we learned in the past century? *International Journal of Behavioral Development*, 24, 129–141.

Tremblay, R. E. (2006). Prevention of youth violence: Why not start at the beginning? *Journal of Abnormal Child Psychology*, 34: 4, 481–487.

Tremblay, R. E., Japel, C., Perusse, D. *et al.* (1999). The search for the age of 'onset' of physical aggression: Rousseau and Bandura revisited. *Criminal Behaviour and Mental Health*, 9, 8–23.

Tremblay, R. E., Nagin, D. S., Seguin, J. R. *et al.* (2004). Physical aggression during early childhood: trajectories and predictors. *Pediatrics*, 114: 1, e43–e50.

Turner, K. M. T. and Sanders, M. R. (2006). Dissemination of evidence-based parenting and family support strategies. *Aggression and Violent Behavior*, 11, 176–193.

Turner, S. and Sloper, P. (1996). Behaviour problems among children with Down's syndrome: prevalence, persistence and parental appraisal. *Journal of Applied Research in Intellectual Disabilities*, 9, 129–144.

Tyrer, F., McGrother, C. W., Thorp, C. F. *et al.* (2006). Physical aggression towards others in adults with learning disabilities: prevalence and associated factors. *Journal of Intellectual Disability Research*, 50, 295–304.

Tyrer, P., Oliver-Africano, P. C., Ahmed, Z. *et al.* (2008). Risperidone, haloperidol, and placebo in the treatment of aggressive challenging behaviour in patients with intellectual disability: a randomised controlled trial. *Lancet*, 371, 57–63.

Ullman, L. and Krasner, L. (1965). *Case Studies in Behavior Modification*. New York: Holt, Rinehart and Winston.

Ungar, M. (2008). Resilience across cultures. *British Journal of Social Work*, 38, 218–235.

Unwin, G. L. and Deb, S. (2008). Use of medication for the management of behavior problems among adults with intellectual disabilities: a clinicians' consensus survey, *American Journal on Mental Retardation*, **113**, 19–31.

Urv, T. K., Zigman, W. B. and Silverman, W. (2008). Maladaptive behaviors related to dementia status in adults with Down syndrome. *American Journal on Mental Retardation*, **113**, 73–86.

US Department of Health and Human Services, A.f.C.a.F. (2010). Head Start Impact Study. Final Report, Washington, DC: US Department of Health and Human Services.

Vaughn, B. J. and Horner, R. H. (1995). Effects of concrete versus verbal choice systems on problem behavior. *AAC: Augmentative and Alternative Communication*, **11**, 89–92.

Vaughn, B. J. and Horner, R. H. (1997). Identifying instructional tasks that occasion problem behaviors and assessing the effects of student versus teacher choice among these tasks. *Journal of Applied Behavior Analysis*, **30**, 299–312.

Vitaro, F. and Tremblay, R. E. (2008). Clarifying and maximising the usefulness of targeted preventative interventions. In M. Rutter, D. Bishop, D. Pine, S. Scott, J. Stevenson, E. Taylor and A. Thapar, eds. *Rutter's Child and Adolescent Psychiatry*. 5th edn. Oxford: Blackwell.

Vollmer, T. R. (1994). The concept of automatic reinforcement: Implications for behavioral research in developmental disabilities. *Research in Developmental Disabilities*, **15**, 187–207.

Vollmer, T. R., Iwata, B. A., Zarcone, J. R., Smith, R. G. and Mazaleski, J. L. (1993). The role of attention in the treatment of attention-maintained self-injurious behavior: noncontingent reinforcement and differential reinforcement of other behavior. *Journal of Applied Behavior Analysis*, **26**, 9–21.

Vollmer, T. R., Marcus, B. A. and Ringdahl, J. E. (1995). Noncontingent escape as a treatment for self-injurious behavior maintained by negative reinforcement. *Journal of Applied Behavior Analysis*, **28**, 15–26.

Vollmer, T. R., Ringdahl, J. E., Roane, H. S. and Marcus, B. A. (1997). Negative side effects of noncontingent reinforcement. *Journal of Applied Behavior Analysis*, **30**, 161–164.

Wacker, D. P., Steege, J. N., Sasso, G. *et al.* (1990). A component analysis of functional communication training across three topographies of severe behavior problems. *Journal of Applied Behavior Analysis*, **23**, 417–429.

Wacker, D. P., Harding, J., Cooper, L. J. *et al.* (1996). The effects of meal scheduling and quantity on problematic behavior. *Journal of Applied Behavior Analysis*, **29**, 79–87.

Wacker, D. P., Berg, W. K., Harding, J. W., Derby, K. M., Asmus, J. M. and Healy, A. (1998). Evaluation and long-term treatment of aberrant behavior displayed by young children with disabilities. *Journal of Developmental and Behavioral Pediatrics*, **19**, 260–266.

Wahler, R. G. (1975). Some structural aspects of deviant child behavior. *Journal of Applied Behavior Analysis*, **8**, 27–42.

Wahler, R. G. (1980). The insular mother: her problems in parent-child treatment. *Journal of Applied Behavior Analysis*, **13**, 207–217.

Wahler, R. G. and Fox, J. J. (1981). Setting events in applied behavior analysis: toward a conceptual and methodological expansion. *Journal of Applied Behavior Analysis*, 14, 327–338.

Wallander, J. L., Dekker, M. C. and Koot, H. M. (2006). Risk factors for psychopathology in children with intellectual disability: a prospective longitudinal population-based study. *Journal of Intellectual Disability Research*, 50, 259–268.

Walsh, P., Emerson, E., Lobb., C. *et al.* (2008). Supported accommodation services for people with intellectual disabilities: a review of models and instruments used to measure quality of life. Dublin: National Disability Authority.

Webster-Stratton, C. and Taylor, T. (2001). Nipping early risk factors in the bud: Preventing substance abuse, delinquency, and violence in adolescence through interventions targeted at young children (0 to 8 years). *Prevention Science*, 2: 3, 165–192.

Webster-Stratton, C., Reid, J. and Stoolmiller, M. (2008). Preventing conduct problems and improving school readiness: evaluation of the Incredible Years Teacher and Child Training Programs in high-risk schools. *Journal of Child Psychology and Psychiatry*, 49, 471–488.

Wehmeyer, M. L., Sands, D. J., Knowlton, E. and Kozleski, E. B. (2002). *Teaching Students with Mental Retardation: Providing Access to the General Curriculum.* Baltimore: Brookes.

Weiss, E. M. (1998). Deadly restraints. *Hartford Courant*, October 11–15.

Weiss, J. A. and Bebko, J. M. (2008). Participation in special Olympics and change in athlete self-concept over 42 months. *Journal on Developmental Disabilities*, 14, 1–8.

Welsh Assembly Government (2005). *Framework for Restrictive Physical Intervention Policy and Practice.* Cardiff: Welsh Assembly Government.

Werner, E. and Smith, R. (1992). *Overcoming the Odds: High Risk Children from Birth to Adulthood.* New York: Cornell University Press.

Werry, J. S., Carlielle, J. and Fitzpatrick, J. (1983). Rhythmic motor activities (stereotypies) in children under five: Etiology and prevalence. *Journal of the American Academy of Child Psychiatry*, 22, 329–336.

Whitaker, S. (1993). The reduction of aggression in people with learning difficulties: a review of psychological methods. *British Journal of Clinical Psychology*, 32, 1–37.

White, M., Adams, J. and Heywood, P. (2009). How and why do interventions that increase health overall widen inequalities within populations? In S. J. Babones, ed. *Social Inequality and Public Health*. Bristol: Policy Press.

Whittingham, K., Sofronoff, K., Sheffield, J. K. and M. R., S. (2009). Stepping Stones Triple P: a randomized controlled trial with parents of a child diagnosed with an Autism Spectrum Disorder. *Journal of Abnormal Child Psychology*, 37, 469–480.

Whittington, J. and Holland, A. J. (2004). *Prader–Willi Syndrome: Development and Manifestations.* Cambridge: Cambridge University Press.

Whittington, R., Lancaster, G., Meehan, C., Lane, S. and Riley, D. (2006). Physical restraint of patients in acute mental health care settings: patient, staff, and environmental factors associated with the use of a horizontal restraint. *Journal of Forensic Psychiatry and Psychology*, 17, 253–265.

Wilding, J., Cornish, K. and Munir, F. (2002). Further delineation of the executive deficit in males with fragile-X syndrome. *Neuropsychologia*, 40, 1343–1349.

Wilkinson, R. G. and Pickett, K. E. (2009). *The Spirit Level: Why More Equal Societies Almost Always Do Better*. London: Penguin.

Willems, E. P. (1974). Behavioral technology and behavioral ecology. *Journal of Applied Behavior Analysis*, 7, 151–165.

Windahl, S. I. (1988). Self injurious behavior in a time perspective. *8th Congress of the International Association for the Scientific Study of Mental Deficiency*, Dublin.

Winslow, C.-E. A. (1920). The untilled fields of public health. *Science*, 23–33.

Winterling, V., Dunlap, G. and O'Neill, R. E. (1987). The influence of task variation on the aberrant behaviors of autistic students. *Education and Treatment of Children*, 10, 105–119.

Wolf, M. M. (1978), Social validity: the case for subjective measurement, or how applied behavior analysis is finding its heart. *Journal of Applied Behavior Analysis*, 11, 203–214.

Wolfensberger, W. (1972). *The Principle of Normalization in Human Services*. Toronto: National Institute of Mental Retardation.

Wolfensberger, W. (1975). *The Origin and Nature of Our Institutional Models*. Syracuse: Human Policy Press.

Woodward, P., Hardy, S. and Joyce, T. (2007). *Keeping it Together: A Guide for Support Staff W with People Whose Behaviour is Challenging*. Brighton: Pavilion.

World Bank (2010). *World Development Report 2010: Development and Climate Change*. Washington: World Bank.

World Health Organization (1992). *The ICD-10 Classification of Mental and Behavioural Disorders: Clinical Descriptions and Diagnostic Guidelines*. Geneva: WHO.

World Health Organization (1996). *ICD-10 Guide for Mental Retardation*. Geneva: World Health Organization.

World Health Organization (2001). *International Classification of Functioning, Disability and Health*. Geneva: World Health Organization.

World Health Organization (2004). *Prevention of Mental Disorders. Effective Interventions and Policy Options*. Geneva: World Health Organization.

World Health Organization (2007). *Atlas: Global Resources for Persons with Intellectual Disabilities*. Geneva: World Health Organization.

World Health Organization (2007a). *International Classification of Functioning, Disability and Health - Children and Youth Version*. ICF-CY, Geneva: World Health Organization.

World Health Organization (2007b). *Achieving Health Equity: From root Causes to Fair Outcomes*. Interim statement, Geneva: World Health Organization.

World Health Organization (2008). *Closing the Gap in a Generation: Health Equity Through Action on the Social Determinants of Health. Final Report of the Commission on the Social Determinants of Health*. Geneva: World Health Organization.

World Health Organization (2008a). *World Health Report 2008: Primary Health Care (Now More Than Ever)*. Geneva: World Health Organization.

World Health Organization (2008b). *mhGAP: Mental Health Gap Action Programme-Scaling up Care for Mental, Neurological, and Substance Use Disorders*. Geneva: World Health Organization.

World Health Organization (2008c). *Closing the gap in a generation: Health Equity Through Action on the Social Determinants of Health. Final Report of the Commission on the Social Determinants of Health*. Geneva: World Health Organization.

Wright, S., Sayer, J., Parr, A., Gray, R., Southern, D. and Gournay, K. (2005). Breakaway and physical restraint training techniques in acute psychiatric nursing: Results from a national survey of training and practice. *Journal of Forensic Psychiatry and Psychology*, **16**, 380–398.

Yeung, W. J., Linver, M. R. and Brooks-Gunn, J. (2002). How money matters for young children's development: parental investment and family processes. *Child Development*, **73**, 1861–1879.

Young, L., Sigafoos, J., Suttie, J., Ashman, A. and Grevell, P. (1998). Deinstitutionalisation of persons with intellectual disabilities: a review of Australian studies. *Journal of Intellectual & Developmental Disability*, **23**, 155–170.

Zarcone, J. R., Rodgers, T. A., Iwata, B. A., Rourke, D. A. and Dorsey, M. F. (1991). Reliability analysis of the motivation assessment scale: a failure to replicate. *Research in Developmental Disabilities*, **12**, 349–360.

Zarcone, J. R., Iwata, B. A., Vollmer, T. R., Jagtiani, S., Smith, R. G. and Mazaleski, J. L. (1993). Extinction of self-injurious escape behavior with and without instructional fading. *Journal of Applied Behavior Analysis*, **26**, 353–360.

Zarola, A. and Leather, P. (2006). Violence and aggression management training for trainers and managers. A national evaluation of the training provision in healthcare settings. Part 1: Research Report, Norwich: HSE Books.

Zimbelman, K. (2005). Instruments for assessing behavioural problems. In J. Hogg and A. Langa, eds. *Assessing Adults with Intellectual Disabilities: A service providers' guide*, Oxford: Blackwell.

Zion, E. and Jenvey, V. B. (2006). Temperament and social behaviour at home and school among typically developing children and children with an intellectually disability. *Journal of Intellectual Disability Research*, **50**, 445–456.

Zubrick, S. R., Northey, K., Silburn, S. R. *et al.* (2005). Prevention of child behavior problems through universal implementation of a group behavioral family intervention. *Prevention Science*, **6**, 287–304.

Index

Printed in the United States
By Bookmasters